LIVING WITH HEART ARRHYTHMIAS AND SURVIVING:

Supraventricular Tachycardia

Also by Barbara O'Shea

We Remember the Day of President Kennedy's Assassination

LIVING WITH HEART ARRHYTHMIAS AND SURVIVING:

Supraventricular Tachycardia

by

Barbara O'Shea

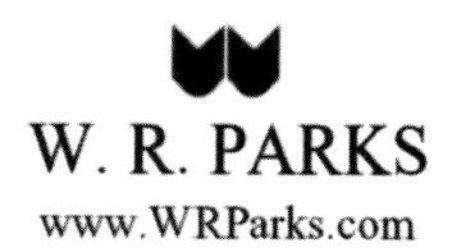

W. R. PARKS
www.WRParks.com

ISBN-13: 978-0-88493-056-3
Library of Congress Control Number:
Published by William R. Parks: www.wrparks.com
Front Cover Artwork by Kelley S. Powers

Dedication

This book is dedicated to the
professional caregivers in my family.

Julia O'Shea, RN
Kelley Powers, OT
Gary Haber, MD
Colleen Powers, SLP
Caroline Powers, RN
Alison Doyle, PT

Contents

LIVING WITH HEART ARRHYTHMIAS AND SURVIVING: Supranventricular Tachycardia

Supraventricular Tachycardia in My Early Years

I was overwhelmed with anxiety when, at age nineteen, my heart suddenly started racing and pounding as I experienced my first episode of supraventricular tachycardia or SVT. "Oh, no," I said, grabbing my sister's arm. "It's happening to *me*!"

Although I felt weak and light-headed, I wasn't surprised. My mother had often experienced the same debilitating exasperation throughout her life, and the condition was believed to run in families. For those in her generation, it seemed nothing much could be done about SVT except to lie down and rest until it passed. I knew of no other remedy, so I followed my mother's example to resolve the situation, and in a few minutes, my heart rate returned to normal. As I recall, my mother's episodes were not long and did not occur often. At the time I didn't realize it, but I have since learned that SVT most commonly occurs in women in their twenties and thirties. My own experience, however, has taught me that the condition can occur throughout life.

During the early years, my episodes were rare, occurring only one or two times per decade. As I grew older, however, these episodes gradually increased in frequency and duration, averaging once a month and lasting anywhere from a half hour to six or seven hours.

One can hardly imagine enduring a rapid pulse rate of 150 to 220 BPM (beats per minute) and feeling overwhelmed with exhaustion as if one had run a marathon. Moreover, one might feel tightness in the throat, dizzy, or light-headed. Syncope (fainting), near fainting, or blacking out can occur. One might also experience shortness of breath or chest pain. Typically, the heart will beat rapidly for reasons unrelated to exercise, fever, or stress. An episode of SVT can come on suddenly and terminate quickly and will usually resolve by itself, but not always. Although some episodes last only a few minutes, others might linger one or two days. Supraventricular tachycardia isn't typically considered life-threatening, but lengthy episodes can be dangerous and should be treated.

Experiencing more frequent and longer episodes of SVT in my later years prompted me to learn all I could about the condition. I soon realized that these rapid palpitations were caused by a flaw in the heart's electrical system, and as a result, my heart could not function properly. Episodes of SVT, as in my case, occur at random and are unpredictable. Keeping a journal can help establish patterns of behavior that might contribute to these episodes. Through my own research, I learned that various medications, such as digoxin or theophylline, could trigger an episode. Decongestants that contain stimulants or stressors, such as nicotine, methamphetamines, cocaine, or too much alcohol, should be avoided. But often one cannot determine what caused the onset. Fortunately, after treatment, or typically on its own, the heart rate returns to normal, or *sinus rhythm*, as it is commonly referred.

Supraventricular tachycardia is not limited to gender or any age or health status. It can occur in healthy people of all ages, including children and adolescents as well as those with or without underlying heart disease. For most people experiencing SVT the heart typically works well, pumping blood throughout the body. Most people with SVT live normal healthy lives without restrictions.

My SVT Intensifies

During the last few years of my teaching career in Youngstown, New York, episodes of SVT occurred more frequently and lasted longer (Figure 1).

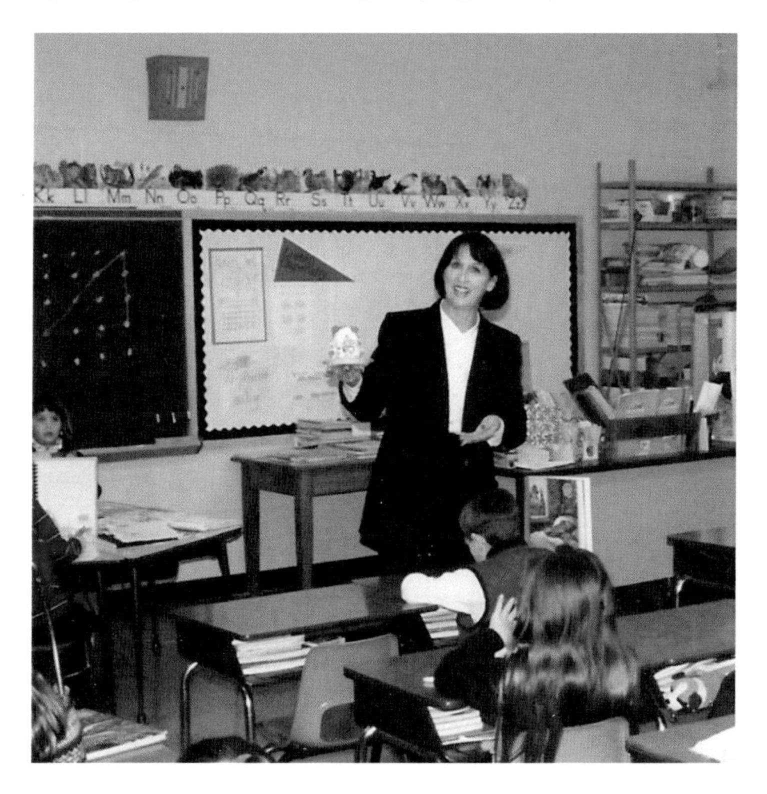

Figure 1. I enjoyed teaching my second-grade students at Lewiston-Porter Central School in Youngstown, NY.

Upon leaving work one fine day in April 1998, I decided that rather than going directly home, I would shop at Niagara Prime Outlets in Niagara Falls. I started down Creek Road, but just beyond the intersection where I would normally turn to go home, however, I experienced an abrupt onset of rapid palpitations. I continued driving, but I suddenly felt like I might faint or blackout, or *even die*, as my surroundings started to fade away.

I pulled onto the shoulder of the road, stopped the car, and shifted into parking gear. I tried to act like nothing was wrong and wondered whether anyone would recognize my car and pull over to help or inquire. I remember feeling as though I might need help, but I regained full consciousness in a moment or two and quickly abandoned the idea of shopping altogether. Shopping requires making decisions and spending money, which is probably why I have often found it to be stressful. Of course, I can only speculate whether it had anything to do with this episode.

My heart rate subsided as I headed east along the familiar, scenic twenty-mile stretch of back roads through Niagara County, passing by the beautiful still waters of Bond Lake. Upon arriving safely home, my heart rate had slowed to 126 bpm, and according to my Omron Hem 609 wrist monitor, my blood pressure was 113/80. I relaxed in a chaise lounge on the deck until the episode, which lasted about an hour, resolved and my heart returned to normal sinus rhythm.

During an episode of SVT, an abnormal electrical impulse starting in the atria triggers the fast heart rate. The heart beats so fast, in fact, that it cannot relax between contractions. The chambers, therefore, might not be strong enough to fill with enough blood to furnish the body's needs at rest or during stress. Because of the ineffective contractions of the heart, the brain does not receive enough blood and oxygen; therefore, one can feel light-headed or dizzy or can blackout, which explains what I had just experienced.

The Heart of the Matter

A month later, on May 28th, an episode of tachycardia occurred upon my arrival at school. At 9:10 a.m., during the announcements after the Pledge of Allegiance over the public-address system, I suddenly began feeling faint and like my heart was palpitating rapidly. I wandered over to my desk where I remained seated for the most part until I walked my students to gym class at ten o'clock.

Fortunately, I had this time free for planning, but instead, I stopped to see the school nurse. I wanted to explain what I was experiencing, and perhaps lie down. First, she checked my heart rate. "Oh, my," she said. "Your pulse is 180!"

Then she fastened the blood pressure cuff to my arm and waited. She became alarmed when she could not get my blood pressure reading. "I'm calling 911," she declared without hesitation. "Go ahead and lie down." She grabbed the phone and dialed the number.

Within a few minutes, the ambulance that would take me to nearby Mount St. Mary's Hospital, pulled up in front of the school. By this time, however, my pulse had returned to a more normal rate of 80, yet my blood pressure was "on the high side," according to the school nurse. "Regardless," she explained, "once you dial 911, the paramedics will follow through."

However, all I had really needed to do during this episode was lay down and rest a while, and my heart would, in time, return to normal sinus rhythm.

Upon arriving at the hospital, I was taken to the emergency department, where the nurses performed extensive blood work and ECG monitoring. All readings were normal. My husband was notified by our school secretary and was present for the doctor to explain to him, "Test results are all normal. I've prescribed medication for relaxing, and your wife is ready to go home. She should rest and sleep most of the remainder of the day."

When I visited my family doctor the next day, he suggested taking a week off work. His nurse hooked me up for an ECG, which measures impulses in the heart through ten small electrodes attached to the skin of the chest, arms, and legs. The doctor showed me a computer printout of those electrical impulses on graph paper. The test also checked for ischemia or poor blood flow. Again, the results were normal. Blood was collected to test for a possible thyroid problem. The doctor scheduled an echocardiogram (sonogram of the heart) for June 8 at the local hospital. Just before leaving the office, the nurse attached me to a 24-hour Holter monitor, an ambulatory electrocardiogram (a portable ECG).

I disregarded my doctor's advice and went to work the next day because SVT episodes are unpredictable, sporadic, and acute rather than chronic. I could be fine one day and have a life-threatening medical emergency the next. Shopping, driving, or sleeping -- it didn't matter what I was doing. I was always at risk for an episode.

I did not experience any noticeable SVT while wearing the Holter monitor. However, the findings did reveal the presence of very rare ventricular premature contractions and supraventricular contractions (Figure 2).

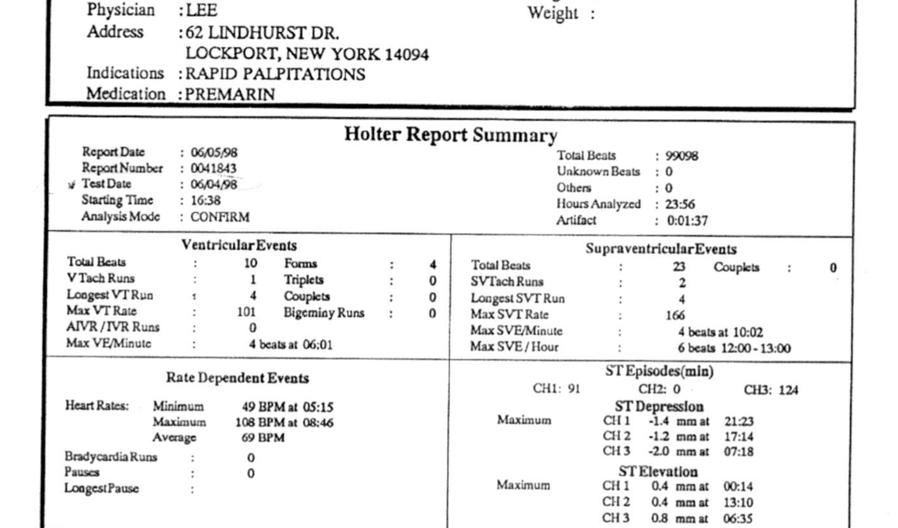

Patient Information

Name	: OSHEA, BARBARA	DOB	: 12/15/38
ID	: 0041843	Age	: 59
Phone	: 433-8609	Height	:
Physician	: LEE	Weight	:
Address	: 62 LINDHURST DR. LOCKPORT, NEW YORK 14094	Sex	: FEMALE
Indications	: RAPID PALPITATIONS		
Medication	: PREMARIN		

Holter Report Summary

Report Date	: 06/05/98	Total Beats	: 99098
Report Number	: 0041843	Unknown Beats	: 0
Test Date	: 06/04/98	Others	: 0
Starting Time	: 16:38	Hours Analyzed	: 23:56
Analysis Mode	: CONFIRM	Artifact	: 0:01:37

Ventricular Events

Total Beats	: 10	Forms	: 4
V Tach Runs	: 1	Triplets	: 0
Longest VT Run	: 4	Couplets	: 0
Max VT Rate	: 101	Bigeminy Runs	: 0
AIVR / IVR Runs	: 0		
Max VE/Minute	: 4 beats at 06:01		

Supraventricular Events

Total Beats	: 23	Couplets	: 0
SVTach Runs	: 2		
Longest SVT Run	: 4		
Max SVT Rate	: 166		
Max SVE/Minute	: 4 beats at 10:02		
Max SVE / Hour	: 6 beats 12:00 - 13:00		

Rate Dependent Events

Heart Rates:	Minimum	49 BPM at 05:15
	Maximum	108 BPM at 08:46
	Average	69 BPM
Bradycardia Runs	:	0
Pauses	:	0
Longest Pause	:	

ST Episodes(min)

CH1: 91 CH2: 0 CH3: 124

		ST Depression	
Maximum	CH 1	-1.4 mm at	21:23
	CH 2	-1.2 mm at	17:14
	CH 3	-2.0 mm at	07:18

		ST Elevation	
Maximum	CH 1	0.4 mm at	00:14
	CH 2	0.4 mm at	13:10
	CH 3	0.8 mm at	06:35

Impressions and Findings

1). Basic rhythm is Normal Sinus Rhythm with average rate 69/bpm.

2). Very rare Premature Ventricular Contractions and Supraventricular Contractions present.

3). Episodes of Ventricular Tachycardia (4-beat run) at 6:01 present. Episode of Supraventricular Tachycardia (4-beat run) at 12:17.

4). No correlated events present with cardiac arrhythmia.

Figure 2. Holter Summary Report

More Testing Includes Echocardiogram

On the morning of June 8, I reported to the hospital at 7:30 a.m. The technician administering the echocardiogram was very knowledgeable and highly skilled and shared what she observed during the test. She explained images we could both see as they appeared on the monitor.

"One cell in the right atrium acts as a manager or messenger," she explained, drawing my attention to it on the screen. "If this cell gets out of sync for some reason, perhaps a skipped beat, the other cells try to compensate by taking over, perhaps resulting in some confusing signals." She told me that my heart appeared very healthy. "You have no evidence of strokes or attacks, and no blockage or chest pain. Any of these symptoms," she added, "would suggest an angiogram as the next step in the testing process." As it was, I didn't need one.

After the echocardiogram, I arrived to work on time. Around 2:25 p.m., however, the "manager" or messenger must have lost focus because my heart started racing again. It had been only eleven days since my last episode. I was sitting at one of the computers in my classroom with Katie, a student, helping her correct spelling errors in a writing sample, a two-page account she had written of a recent trip to Florida. Some students were working independently on a spelling lesson, and a few others had left the room for remedial math instruction.

As usual, I immediately began feeling faint, with major blood flow drawn to my heart. I thought about the "manager" analogy the technician had described to me earlier in the day, which seemed to help slow my heart rate. Within a few minutes, my heart returned to a normal sinus rhythm. Katie's mom picked her up at three o'clock and asked how I was doing. After explaining what had happened, she told me she had a prolapsed valve, which can cause the same symptoms I experience. My echocardiogram, however, did not reveal any valve issues (Figure 3).

Echocardiography

IP ______ OP X

Report

Test Date 6/08/98

Name: O'SHEA, BARBARA Age: 59 DOB: 12/15/38 ID # 41843

Requesting MD LEE Ht.: 5'6" Wt.: 133 BSA 1.68 Tape #: S-185

Clinical Information: Palpitations, chest pain, mitral valve prolapse.

Technical Limitations: ______

2D/M-Mode Measurements (Reference: *Echocardiography*, 5th Edition by Feigenbaum, 1994)					
Site	Results	Normals	Site	Results	Normals
Aorta	2.7	2.0 - 3.7 cm	IVS (Diastole)	0.9	0.6 - 1.1 cm
L.A. (Systole)	4.0	1.9 - 4.0 cm	IVS (Systole)	1.3	Variable
A.C. Excursion	1.5	1.5 - 2.6 cm	LVPW (Diastole)	0.6	0.6 - 1.1 cm
RVID	normal	0.9 - 2.6 cm	LVPW (Systole)	1.4	Variable
LVID (Diastole)	5.1	3.5 - 5.7 cm	Fractional Shortening	0.40	0.28 - 0.41
LVID (Systole)	3.0	Variable	LV Function	70%	>55%

IMPRESSION:

AV: Structure, motility valve opening and closure is normal.
AO: Root is normal.
MV: Structure, motility valve opening and closure is normal. No evidence of prolapse.
LA: Size is at the upper limits of normal. No thrombus.
LV: Size is normal. Good wall motion. Ejection fraction is 70%.
RA: Size is normal.
RV: Size is normal. No pericardial effusion.

DOPPLER EXAM: MILD MITRAL REGURGITATION. FLOW ACROSS THE AV, TRICUSPID, PULMONARY VALVE NORMAL.

CONCLUSION:

1. LV size and systolic function is normal. Ejection fraction is 70%.
2. LA size is at the upper limits of normal. No thrombus.
3. RA, RV chamber size is normal.
4. No evidence of mitral valve prolapse.
5. Mild mitral regurgitation.

Figure 3. Echocardiography Report

In Anticipation of Upcoming Events

During that summer, I experienced two brief episodes of SVT, both of which occurred in the morning upon awakening. Therefore, I wasn't surprised when, on September 9, 1998—the first day of school—a brief episode occurred again upon awakening. Coincidentally, at the time, I had been thinking about the previous two episodes. Fortunately, conversion occurred quickly, and I was able to drive to work. I enjoyed meeting my new second-grade class of eight boys and twelve girls and a full-time aide, Joan, who was assigned to assist one of my students with special needs. We played a get-acquainted game called Friendship Bingo, which took up the entire morning. It was a half day for students, so they were dismissed at noon. I had felt fine all morning, so I stayed in the afternoon and worked with Joan, who assisted me in designing a pamphlet using Microsoft Word.

I had begun to wonder whether important upcoming events could trigger the onset of an episode of SVT. The first day of a new school year, for example, was much like starting any new job. Thinking about it could cause anxiety and stress and restless nights as I realized that those warm, sunny days of leisure and relaxation were over, and it was back to work. When we were kids, most of us started the school year with a new pair of shoes. As an adult, I was confronted with a classroom comprised of twenty-five unfamiliar faces with a wide range of personalities, individual differences, learning styles, and special needs.

No wonder during the week or two before school began in September, I had dreams just short of nightmares, as I imagine many teachers probably do, in anticipation of the start of a new school year. These dreams were typically filled with dreadful situations wherein everything possible, even the simplest tasks, went awry. I recall in one such dream standing in front of the class teaching a lesson on the first day when it suddenly occurred to me that I hadn't stopped in the office to pick up my schedule specifying what time and on which days my students had art, gym, or music. I wondered whether it was that time, or if they had missed their special altogether. Then I realized that I hadn't even taken attendance or lunch count.

I should note that although I had many episodes of SVT during the year 1999, unfortunately, I have no records, as I did not keep a journal during that time.

Again, it wasn't uncommon for me to wake up some mornings with an episode of tachycardia arrhythmia and *possible* atrial fibrillation, also known as A-Fib, which can be debilitating. On March 3, 2000, my husband and I traveled to Binghamton, New York, his hometown, to attend the Annual St. Patrick's Day Parade the next day. It was an important day in my life, which I had been anxiously awaiting.

On the morning of the parade, however, I couldn't even make it downstairs to the hotel restaurant for breakfast with my husband and our friends, Mary Kay and Kevin, who had met us in Binghamton. I tried getting dressed a few times, but each time, I felt exasperated and incapacitated by the lack of energy. I was too weak to do anything but lie down and collapse on the bed. I felt pressure on my chest and was light-headed and faint. My pulse was so weak it was impossible to detect. It seemed like the worst episode of my life, which at the time I thought might have been triggered by caffeine.

After dinner the previous evening, I had made the mistake of drinking two cups of regular coffee, something I hadn't done in a few months. I had started drinking green tea concentrate about a month prior and avoided regular coffee with caffeine or any coffee beyond the usual two cups at breakfast. I have since learned, however, that moderate amounts of caffeine are not likely to trigger tachycardia. Most people do not have to avoid caffeinated coffee, tea, soft drinks, or chocolate.

In addition, I learned that one *can* reduce the risk of having an episode of SVT by avoiding certain other stimulants such as nicotine, methamphetamines, cocaine, and alcohol. Decongestants that contain stimulants should be avoided, too, such as oxymetazoline (Afrin), pseudoephedrine (Sudafed), and diet pills, pep pills, and ephedrine. By keeping a diary or journal, one might be able to identify stressors.

Fear of not being able to attend the parade weighed heavily on my mind throughout this episode. About mid-morning, however, I finally finished getting dressed and ready for breakfast. My heart rate seemed closer to normal. I called Mary Kay, who was in her room reading a book, and she was happy to go down and keep me company while I munched on a toasted English muffin covered with a smudge of strawberry jelly, and instead of the usual coffee, a glass of pineapple juice. This episode had lasted about two-and-a-half hours.

We finally arrived at the St. Patrick's Day Parade, where I ultimately succeeded in reaching my goal: shaking hands with the potential next president of the United States, Texas Governor George W. Bush. We had been standing five rows deep from the curb, when I managed to stoop, wiggle, and twist my way through the crowd as he marched down Court Street in the parade alongside Governor George Pataki of New York. My husband was not a Republican, or he would have squirmed his way along with me to the front and taken a picture of us (Figures 4 and 5).

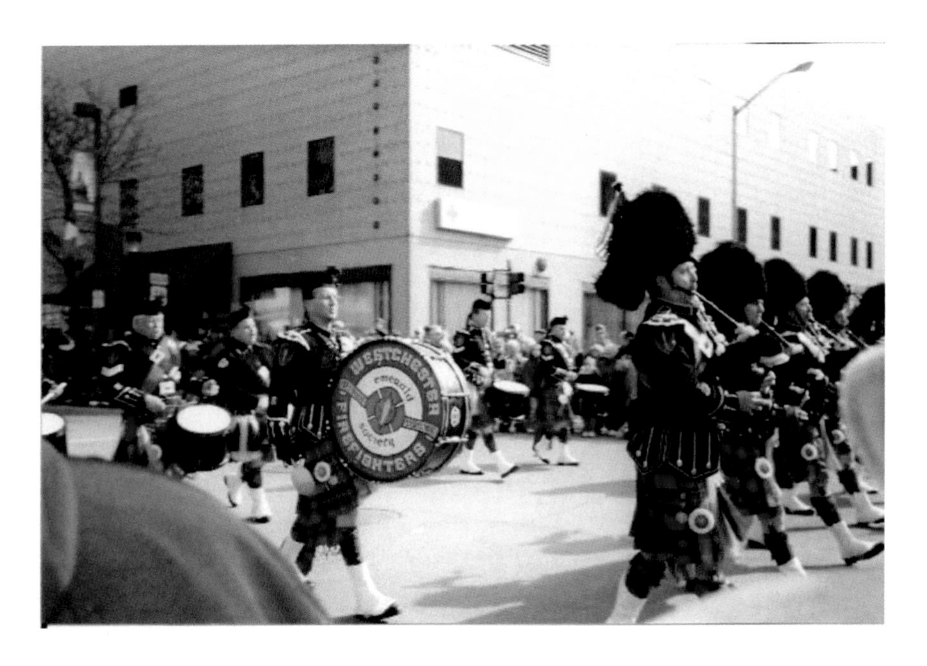

Figure 4. St. Patrick's Day Parade with drum and bugle corps, elected officials, and high school bands marching down Court Street.

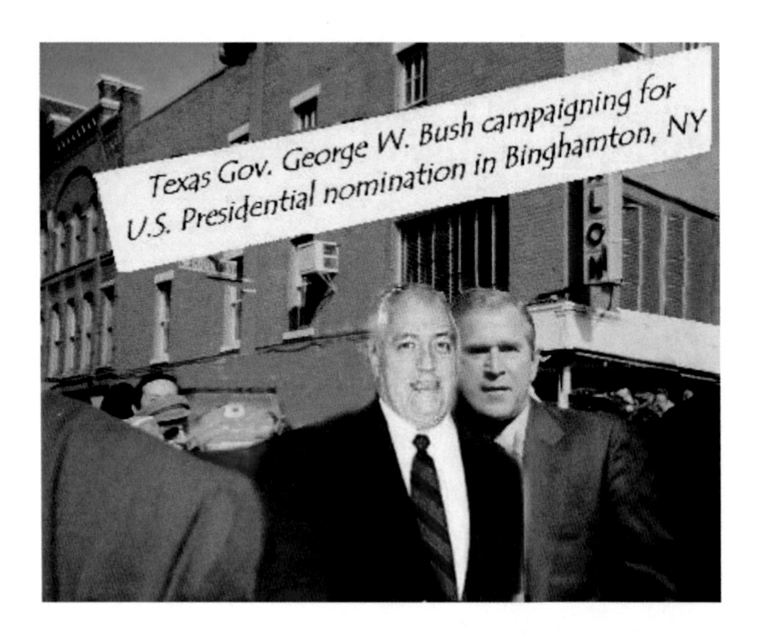

Figure 5. I snapped a picture of Texas Governor George W. Bush (right) as he marched down Court Street in Binghamton, New York.

I wondered whether stress associated with an unsolicited task or event might trigger an episode of tachycardia. I certainly did feel somewhat stressed when my husband asked the night before if I would drive after the parade the next day from Binghamton to Harrisburg, Pennsylvania. A year ago, I had experienced a tense, hectic drive down I-81 South in the Scranton–Wilkes Barre area because of massive road construction, signs, lane shifts, and heavy traffic. Abysmal! I wanted to switch drivers at that time, but I could find no place to pull off the road. Admittedly, I was not looking forward to driving that route again and hoped construction had ended. Fortunately, it had, and it was an easy drive.

Another Travel Episode of Tachycardia

Six weeks later, on April 16, I awakened at four o'clock in the morning thinking about the volatile stock market when I suddenly experienced another episode of cardiac arrhythmia or SVT. My husband and I were overnighting at the Sheraton Four Points Hotel on Lake Erie in Dunkirk, New York, in route from an enlightening trip to Charlottesville, Virginia, and Monticello, home of Thomas Jefferson.

During our visit to Charlottesville, we had enjoyed a walking tour of the plantation at Monticello. We learned about the implementation of slavery and the names of many of Jefferson's slaves, including Sally Hemings, whom he had summoned to France to assist in rearing his two daughters while he was a minister to France for five years. According to our tour guide, Thomas Jefferson was a self-taught architect who designed his historic home. His children and grandchildren also lived there, and his aunt taught them to read and write. They, in turn, taught some of the slave children. Even though he opposed slavery, Jefferson owned about 135 slaves. We also visited Jefferson's grave, located nearby on his fifty-acre property, where his descendants are also buried (Figures 6 and 7).

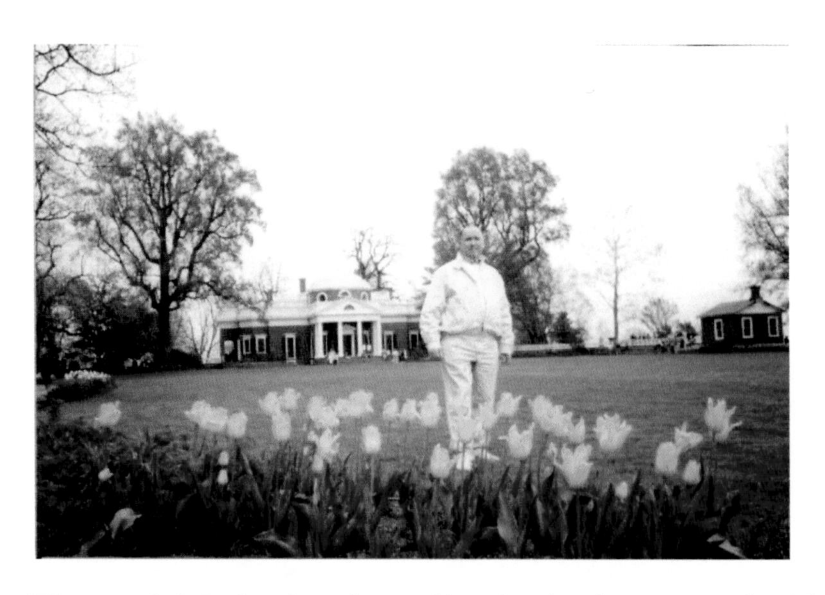

Figure 6. My husband standing in the foreground with Thomas Jefferson's home in the background.

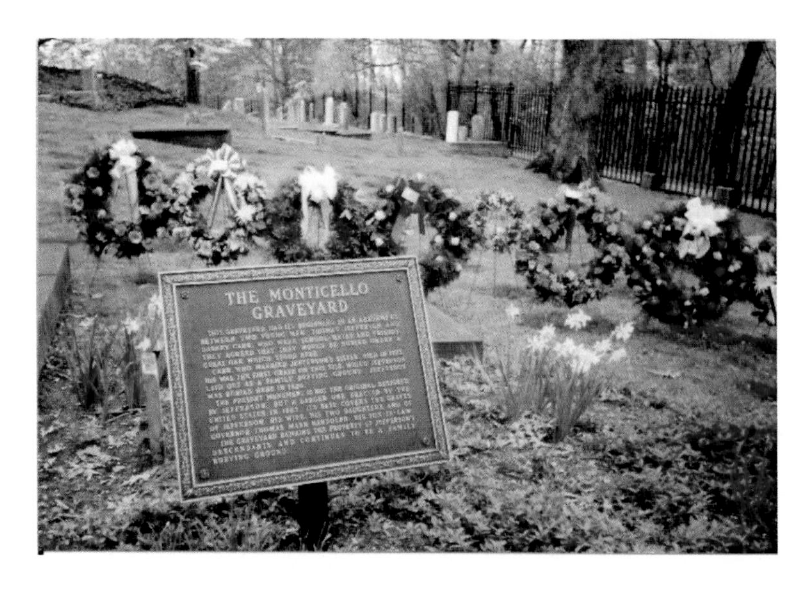

Figure 7. The site where Thomas Jefferson and his family are buried at Monticello.

In addition to serving as the third president of the United States, Thomas Jefferson was the lead author of the Declaration of Independence, the first secretary of state, the second vice president, minister to France, an architect, and a writer.

Stopping in Dunkirk, New York, for an overnight provided a great opportunity for me to revisit the city where I was born and raised. I enjoyed returning here every summer, especially to attend the fabulous Fourth of July fireworks display set off at the foot of the pier near the hotel. But the city that once had a population of 16,000 now had only 11,000 residents. It was stressful to think about the loss of jobs that caused the exodus.

Despite having an episode of SVT there in the middle of the night, I was able to get some sleep intermittently. However, the rapid heart rate and feelings of exhaustion did not fully subside until I arrived downstairs in the beautiful Crow's Nest restaurant for breakfast that morning. It was about ten o'clock, very much like the previous episode in Binghamton in terms of the time of day and setting. Tom enjoyed the full buffet, but I could only eat a piece of toast and drink a cup of decaffeinated coffee. The episode lasted about six hours.

Skipped Heartbeat and Sudden Death Concerns

About two months later, our daughter Susan, son-in-law Mike Powers, and their girls were visiting us for the weekend at our home in Lockport, New York. Tom, a staunch Democrat, invited Mike to join him for brunch at the Ramada Inn in Niagara Falls, New York, a twenty-mile jaunt from our home. Hilary Clinton (then the first lady) was running for New York State Senate and was a scheduled guest speaker at this event in early July. Tom and Mike seized the opportunity to shake hands with her, introducing themselves and exchanging a few words.

Early the next morning, Susan and her family departed for their return trip to Harrisburg, the state capital of Pennsylvania. They took along Susan's childhood maple desk that we had bequeathed to our granddaughter, Colleen, on her eighth birthday.

I felt fine until shortly after three o'clock, just about the time they arrived home when an episode of rapid palpitations occurred. It worried me considerably because I realized that this condition can cause the heart to fill with blood and can result in a blackout due to the lack of blood and oxygen in the brain. I had learned that a skipped heartbeat or a disruption in the normal functioning of the electrical conduction system triggers these episodes. A skipped heartbeat can cause sudden death. However, that day's episode lasted only an hour, after which I was feeling fine and ready to go grocery shopping at Tops Super Market for a few items.

That was the first episode in July, but two more were on the horizon. Exactly three weeks later, on July 23, shortly after I had awakened that morning, I experienced a debilitating episode of SVT that lasted about eight hours. As we were leaving Sunday Mass at our church, I mentioned to Tom that the rapid palpitations that had started earlier that morning had not yet subsided. We debated going to the emergency department at our local hospital but decided to go straight home. Usually, it's not necessary to go to the emergency department, but everyone needs to make their own call depending on their individual circumstances. Unfortunately, one doesn't know at what moment an episode will subside – or begin, for that matter.

Upon arriving home and eating a hearty spinach salad, I began feeling better, although I could not get a blood pressure reading, only ERROR, probably because my heart was still racing at 165 bpm. Finally, after lying down and resting a while, at about five o'clock the readings returned to normal: blood pressure, 105/78 and heart rate, 75.

The third episode in July occurred the very next day. Working late on my computer and scanner project at home and encountering some unexpected technical problems and related stress, I encountered a moment of *terror*, nearly blacking out as a result of some sort of irregular or skipped heartbeat. However, rapid palpitations did not follow. Instead, it felt like my heart had stopped beating altogether. I remembered hearing that a skipped heartbeat can cause sudden death, and that's exactly what I believed was happening. I tried coughing hard a few times and pounding on my chest, and I finally managed to pull myself together. It was the second time this had happened to me. It was a very frightening experience, which prompted me to call my doctor's office the next morning to schedule an appointment.

Follow-up with My Doctor and a Cardiologist and More Testing

Three days later, on July 27, I met with my family doctor (Internal Medicine) at his office concerning my frequent episodes of SVT and more importantly, to discuss what had just happened. I was eager to explain what I had experienced three days earlier. He listened intently to my concerns as he fastened the blood pressure cuff to my forearm. The reading fell within my normal range, 105/65, which he thought was fine. I spent about twenty minutes describing in detail my lifelong episodes of SVT. After hearing all I had to say, he referred me to a local cardiologist, who he would call and explain everything. After that, I would get a call from the cardiologist's office to set up an appointment.

Finally, the day of my appointment with the cardiologist arrived: September 26, 2000. Although it was scheduled for 10:45 a.m., it wasn't until 11:45 that I met with the doctor for consultation regarding the increased frequency and duration of my episodes of cardiac arrhythmia. His nurse had completed a workup of my history and administered an ECG (Figure 8).

RE: BARBARA OSHEA
DOB: 12/15/38
Patient was seen in the office on 9/26/00.

REASON FOR CONSULTATION: Patient with a history of frequent palpitations, cardiac arrhythmia.

HISTORY: Patient is a 61-year-old retired teacher with a history of "rapid palpitations" all my life. Palpitations are more frequent the last few months lasting 2-6 hours. Patient complains of "feeling weak and pulses weak". She denies any dizziness or diaphoresis. No loss of consciousness. No nausea. No vomiting.

REVIEW OF SYSTEMS: Frequent episodes of palpitations and weak feeling. No loss of consciousness. Denies history of chest pain.
No nausea, vomiting, constipation, or diarrhea. No urinary complaints.
No headache. No blurred vision. No recent cough, fever or chills.
Appetite has been normal. Patient has no difficulty with sleep.

CARDIAC WORK-UP: Patient's cardiac work-up done in the past:
2D echo done 6/98 revealed normal LV function.
ETT with Cardiolite 8/95. No evidence of ischemia.
24 hour Holter monitor revealed PVCs, PACs and ventricular tachycardia.
The 24 hour Holter was done 6/06/98.

PHYSICAL EXAMINATION: Well-built and nourished white female.
Height 5'5". Weight 135 lbs. BP 130/86. Heart rate of 72. Respirations 16.
JVP normal.
Carotids felt without bruit.
Peripheral pulses are well-felt and equal.
CHEST: Symmetrical, movements normal.
LUNGS: Clear to percussion & auscultation. No rhonchi or rales heard.
CARDIOVASCULAR: S1, S2 normal. No murmur or rub heard.
ABDOMEN: Soft, nontender. No mass. Bowel sounds are normal.

EKG: Normal sinus rhythm, no acute changes.

CLINICAL IMPRESSION: Sixty-one-year-old white female with cardiac arrhythmia, SVT and ventricular tachycardia, symptomatic, and normal LV function.

PLAN OF TREATMENT: Will check all lab data. Report 2D echo and carotid Doppler. Repeat ETT with Cardiolite to assess coronary status. Patient subsequently had all her cardiac work-up done.

Repeat 2D echo 9/26/00; LV size and function normal. EF is 65%. LA size upper limit of normal. No thrombus.
ETT with Cardiolite done at LMH; Good exercise tolerance. No evidence of ischemia.
Recent 24 hour Holter monitor done 10/17/00; Frequent episodes of SVT, frequent PVCs, couplets.

Figure 8. My patient history for the cardiologist

When I arrived home an hour later, I grabbed a banana for lunch and drove over to the Emmett Belknap Middle School track for a two-mile roller blading workout on the paved area behind the fence that encircled the track (Figure 9).

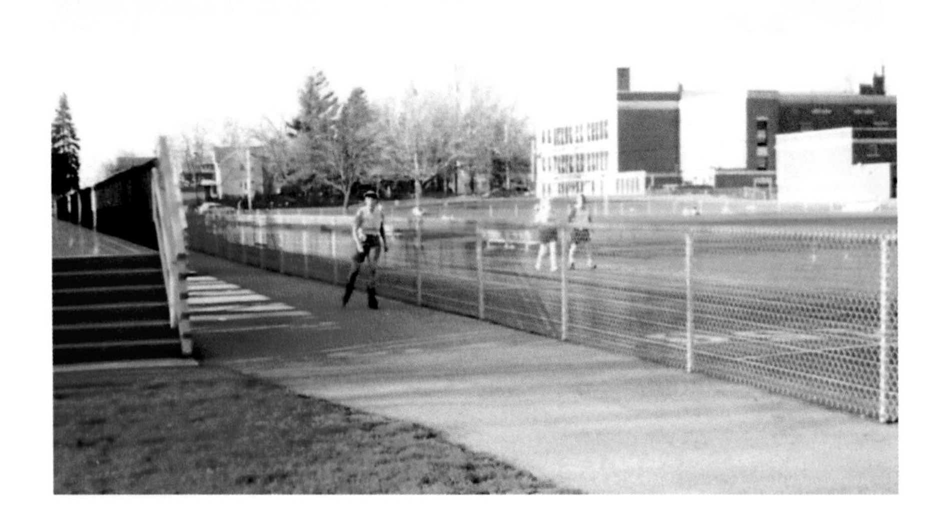

Figure 9. After my morning session with the cardiologist, I energized myself with two miles of rollerblading.

At 2:15 p.m., after rollerblading, I returned to the cardiologist's office for an echocardiogram, a sonogram of the vessels in my neck. All results were normal (Figure 10).

ECHOCARDIOGRAPHY REPORT

Patient: Barbara O'shea **DOB:** 12/15/38
* **Date Of Study:** 9/26/00

AGE: 61
HT: 5'5"
WT: 135
BSA: 1.66

64 DAVISON COURT
LOCKPORT, NY 14094
TEL. 433-1562

Referring Physician: **Tape No.** **N-35**
Clinical Information: Palpitations, dizziness, chest pain

REPORT:

AV: Structure, motility, valve opening and closure is normal.
AO: Aortic root appears normal.
MV: Structure, motility, valve opening and closure is normal. No evidence for prolapse seen.
LA: Size upper limit of normal. No thrombus.
LV: Size, systolic function normal. EF is 65%.
RA: Size normal.
RV: Size normal.
No pericardial effusion.

DOPPLER EXAM: Trace mitral regurgitation.
Flow across the remaining valves is normal.

CONCLUSION:

1. **LV SIZE, SYSTOLIC FUNCTION NORMAL. EF IS 65%.**
2. **LA SIZE UPPER LIMIT OF NORMAL. NO THROMBUS.**
3. **RA, RV CHAMBER SIZE NORMAL.**
4. **TRACE MITRAL REGURGITATION.**

2D/M-Mode Measurements (Reference: Echocardiography, 5th Edition by Feigenbaum, 1994)

Site	Results	Normals	Site	Results	Normals
Aorta	3.33	2.0-3.7 cm.	IVS (Diastole)	0.93	0.6-1.1 cm.
L.A. (Systole)	4.00	1.9-4.0 cm.	IVS (Systole)	1.27	Variable
A.C. Excursion	1.93	1.5-2.6 cm.	LVPW (Diastole)	0.87	0.6-1.1 cm.
RVID	Normal	0.9-2.6 cm.	LVPW (Systole)	1.67	Variable
LVID (Diastole)	3.93	3.5-5.7 cm.	Fractional Shortening	0.34	0.28-0.41
LVID (Systole)	2.60	Variable	LV Function	65%	>55%

Figure 10. Echocardiography report

Without eating a single morsel of food after midnight, I reported to the Lockport Memorial Hospital registration desk on Monday, October 16, at 7:30 a.m. I was directed to the Cardiology Department on the third floor for a stress test. After monitoring a blood pressure reading of 110/70, the registered nurse attached an intravenous (IV) catheter into my right arm near the top of my wrist, after which I stepped on a treadmill and started walking.

During this time, I was able to gaze out the window and watch the Washington Hunt Elementary School teachers pull into their parking places in the school lot. The speed and incline of the treadmill increased every three minutes.

After about ten minutes, I was asked if I walked regularly. "Yes, on the treadmill," I replied, "but I prefer rollerblading as I find it more therapeutic and relaxing."

When I finally stepped off the treadmill, having reached a speed of 4.2 mph, my pulse was clocked at 146 bpm and my blood pressure reading was 160/70.
"You did well," the cardiologist told me. "However, you had a few skipped heartbeats, especially near the end."
I wasn't surprised. "I'll call my office to set up an appointment for you to come in tomorrow to attach a 24-hour Holter monitor," he added, "so that I can tell what is happening while you sleep" (Figure 11).

CARDIAC STRESS LABORATORY

EXERCISE TREADMILL TESTING REPORT

Patient: **O'SHEA, Barbara** Medical Record #: 41843 Date: 10/16/2000

Referring Physician:

HT: 5'6" WT: AGE: 61 TEST TYPE: Scan

1. Reason for study: Palpitations, chest pain
2. Cardiac drugs: None
   Allergies: NKA
3. History: Cardiac arrhythmia
   Risk factors: Family history of CAD and arrhythmia
4. Treadmill: Protocol: Bruce Minutes: 11 METs: 12
5. Reason for stopping exercise: Fatigue
6. Heart rate: Rest: 63 Exercise: 146 Predicted Maximal: 92%
7. Blood Pressure: Rest: 110/70 Exercise: 160/70
8. Double Product: Rest: 6930 Exercise: 23,360
9. Arrhythmia: Rest: None
   During Exercise: Rare PVC
   After Exercise: Rare PVC
10. ECG changes: Rest: None
    During Exercise: None
    After Exercise: None
11. INTERPRETATIONS:

	NORMAL	ABNORMAL	BORDERLINE
A. ST changes	X		
B. HR response	X		
C. BP response	X		
D. Work capacity	X		

12. **Comments**: Patient exercised on a Bruce protocol for 11 minutes, achieving a MET level of 12, a double product of 23,360 and a peak heart rate of 146, which is 92% of predicted maximum for her age. Exercise was terminated because of fatigue.

    No chest pain, no ischemic changes with exercise.

    Rare PVCs with exercise and post exercise.

    Myocardial scan post exercise, results pending.

IMPRESSION: ETT NEGATIVE FOR ISCHEMIA AT A GOOD WORKLOAD, 12 METS. RARE PVC WITH EXERCISE, PATIENT ASYMPTOMATIC.

Figure 11. Exercise treadmill stress test report

After the stress test, I drove home, ate breakfast, and returned to Lockport Memorial Hospital Nuclear Medicine Department for twenty-five minutes of myocardial perfusion imaging. Typically, a small amount of a clear radioactive diagnostic liquid is injected into the bloodstream via an IV catheter and taken up to the heart muscle. Then a special camera takes pictures. Doctors can determine the blood flow through the heart and additional structural information regarding the heart (Figure 12).

Nuclear Medicine Consultation Report

Patient's Name: O'SHEA, Barbara

62 Lindhurst Drive Lockport, NY
Study: Exercise Myocardial Images (SPECT)
Resting Myocardial Images (SPECT)
Gated SPECT Images

Date: 10/16/00 & 10/17/00
Code No: EM-00-10-2027
RM-00-10-2027
GS-00-10-2041

CLINICAL HISTORY: 61 year old white female was referred for Stress Myocardial Perfusion scan to evaluate her complaint of palpitations. Patient risk factors include positive family history for CAD. She was exercised on a treadmill using Bruce Protocol which was terminated because of fatigue after 11 minutes at the end workload of 13 METS. Peak heart rate achieved was 146 minute (92% predicted maximum). Patient is 5'6" in height.

TECHNIQUE: SPECT myocardial images were obtained on 2 different days approximately 1-2 hours following intravenous injection of 16.5 mCi Tc-SESTAMIBI (Cardiolite) and 17.0 mCi Tc-TETROFOSMIN (Myoview) at peak exercise and at rest. SPECT myocardial images were displayed in the horizontal short, horizontal long and vertical long axes slices. Planar images were also obtained in the anterior view. Post-stress gated SPECT study was obtained. Images, wall motion study, systolic wall thickening were analyzed and LV function (LVEF) was calculated.

SCINTIGRAPHIC FINDINGS: The studies demonstrate normal perfusion pattern to the LV myocardium. There are no fixed or reversible perfusion defects. The size of the left ventricle is normal. The post-stress gated SPECT study shows normal wall motion & systolic wall thickening of the left ventricle. The global LV function is normal with LVEF of 66%.

IMPRESSION: NORMAL TOMOGRAPHIC (SPECT) STRESS & RESTING MYOCARDIAL PERFUSION IMAGES. THE STUDIES DEMONSTRATE NO EVIDENCE FOR THE PRESENCE OF STRESS INDUCED MYOCARDIAL ISCHEMIA AT THE END WORKLOAD OF 13 METS.

POST-STRESS GATED SPECT MYOCARDIAL PERFUSION SCAN DEMONSTRATES NORMAL WALL MOTION & SYSTOLIC WALL THICKENING OF THE LV. THE GLOBAL LV FUNCTION IS NORMAL WITH LVEF OF 66%.

Figure 12. Nuclear medicine consultation report

Holter Monitor and Diagnostic Evidence

A few days later, on Friday, October 20, my cardiologist's office called asking me to come in to review my Holter test results. Fortunately, a two-hour episode of SVT had occurred between 8:15 and 10:15 p.m., which the monitor recorded, and this provided the doctor with a documented diagnosis of a rhythm typical of *atrioventricular (AV) nodal re-entrant paroxysmal SVT (PSVT)*; at a rate of about 190 bpm that converted to atrial fibrillation with aberrant conduction, and then sinus rhythm subsequently resumed.

According to the cardiologist, episodes of PSVT (paroxysmal supraventricular tachycardia) originate from a single aorta focus. An electrical loop develops in the region of the AV node, causing the impulse to move in a continuous circle. It takes very little time to conduct around this loop, which causes a continuous "re-entering" into areas already passed and results in a rapid heart rate. He also explained that most people have only one source in the electrical-conductive system to generate a heartbeat, but that I *might* have more than one. Nevertheless, I have a strong, healthy heart (Figures 13 and 14).

24 HOUR HOLTER MONITOR

Patient: **Barbara Oshea** Date: **10/17/00**
ID #: 014-115
Age: 61 yrs.

Reason For Test: Palpitations, cardiac arrhythmia.

Interpretation:

1. **NORMAL SINUS RHYTHM, AVERAGE HEART RATE IS 81/MIN.**
2. **SINUS BRADYCARDIA, RATE OF 47/MIN. AT 4:35 AM.**
3. **MAXIMUM HEART RATE IS 155-160/MIN., 132/MIN. AT 3:38 PM.**
4. **FREQUENT EPISODES OF SUPRAVENTRICULAR TACHYCARDIA WITH HEART RATE OF 176/MIN., 9:07 PM., 9:08 PM., 9:30 PM., 9:35 PM., 9:47 PM.**
5. **VENTRICULAR ECTOPY, COUPLETS.**
6. **PATIENT IS SYMPTOMATIC.**

Figure 13. Holter monitor report, October 17, 2000

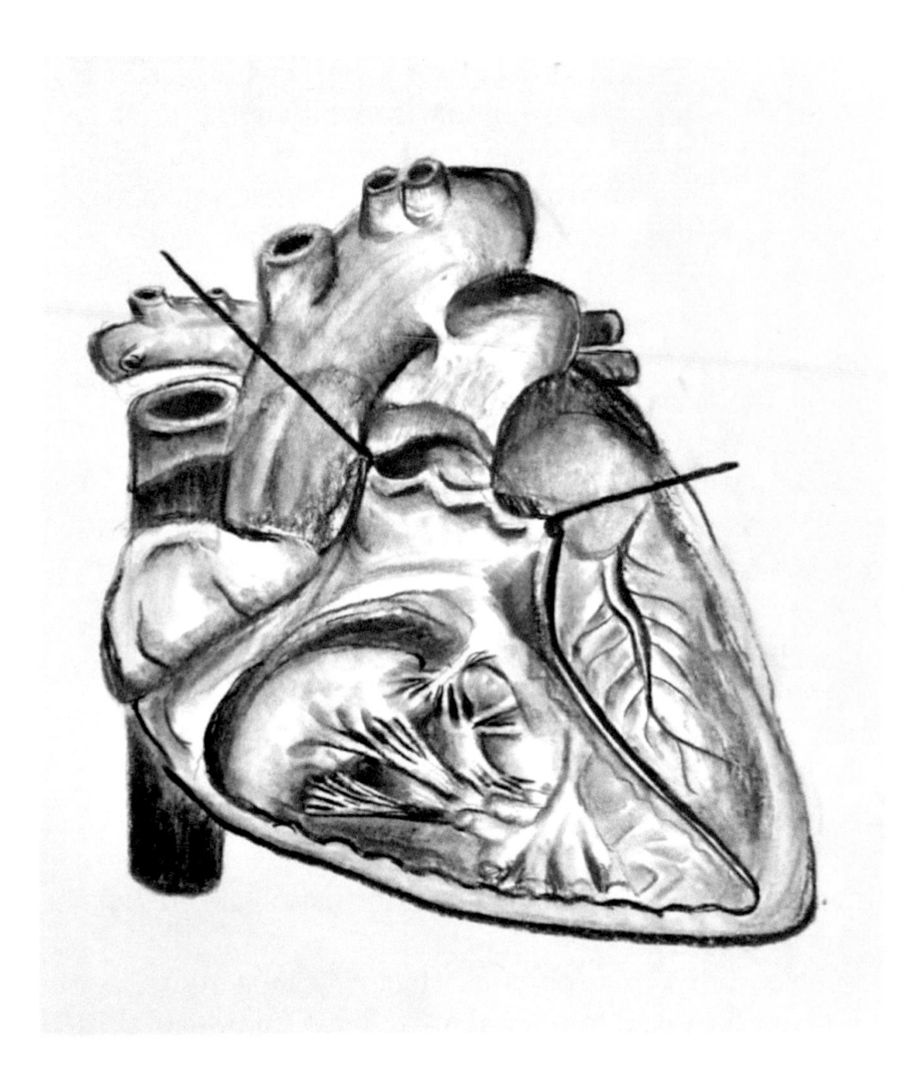

Figure 14. Image of heart. Lines indicate a top layer of this heart being pulled back, so deeper layers are visible. Illustrated by Kelley S. Powers, copyright © 2019

How Can You Mend a Broken Heart?

Before I left his office, the cardiologist prescribed me a beta-blocker, ten milligrams Inderal three times a day, and he told me these episodes would not occur again. He explained that beta-blockers slow the heart rate and therefore decrease the force with which the heart muscle contracts, thereby limiting how narrow the blood vessels become. Beta-blockers are usually prescribed to manage abnormal heart rhythms, but they have side effects, too. Slowing the heart rate relieves stress on the heart, but it can make one feel tired, fatigued, or drowsy. I've since learned they are useful in protecting the heart from a second heart attack after a first attack, as in my brother-in-law's case.

The most common forms of SVT are (1) atrioventricular nodal re-entrant tachycardia (AVNRT), which is most common in adults, accounting for 50-60 percent of all SVT; (2) atrioventricular reciprocating tachycardia (AVRT), which is more common in children; and (3) atrial tachycardia (AT), which is least common. Other types of SVT include atrial fibrillation and flutter.

Heart rhythm problems affect people in all walks of life. I was surprised to learn that some well-known entertainers, athletes, politicians, authors, etc. suffer from these conditions, as well.

In 2011, singer and songwriter Barry Manilow revealed his own experiences with episodes of A-Fib (atrial fibrillation) and tachycardia and has been treated with medication to manage heart rhythm disorders. President George H. W. Bush encountered shortness of breath and tightness in the chest while jogging at Camp David in 1991 and was diagnosed with A-Fib. It was caused by hyperthyroidism or an overactive thyroid gland, and drug therapy was used to return his heart to normal sinus rhythm. Larry Bird, the Boston Celtics basketball star, was also diagnosed with A-Fib, which he encountered during the off-season and after retiring in 1992. A few years later, his episodes had increased in frequency, occurring almost every three months, and he has since been treated with medication. Singer Elton John collapsed during a flight and subsequently required a pacemaker in 1999, which allowed him to continue to perform. Miley Cyrus, former Disney Channel teen star, suffered tachycardia and shortness of breath, lightheadedness, and fainting. Vice President Joseph Biden was diagnosed with atrial fibrillation in 2003 after gall bladder surgery. Sleep apnea was said to have triggered the episode in his case, and he was advised to exercise more and drink less coffee.

On Monday, November 6, I had an appointment with a local electrophysiologist (one who specializes in cardiac arrhythmias) in Buffalo, New York. After reviewing the printout of my recent twenty-four-hour Holter monitor reading (see Figure 13), he explained a procedure used effectively for about the past ten years called a catheter or radiofrequency ablation, which offers a *cure* for SVT and is especially recommended for those with persistent and recurrent episodes.

"The procedure has a 98 percent success rate of curing the condition and with low risk," he explained. "While the patient is semi-conscious, a thin wire is threaded into the numbed groin and up through the veins and into the heart where it identifies the source of the problem, ablates or destroys it, and accelerates it again to see if the problem has been corrected. Typically, a lesion five millimeters in depth is enough to destroy the full thickness of the atrial myocardium in that location."

The electrophysiologist explained the other option, that is, living with lifelong and relatively unpredictable recurrences of tachycardia. "Certainly," he said, "episodes might be better tolerated and less frequent by using a variety of alternative drugs in addition to Inderal, but it would not resolve or cure the problem." He explained that various drugs may chemically interrupt conduction in the loop. "Of course, if you prefer drug therapy," he added, "I would increase the Inderal and add flecainide if needed."

I was not a huge fan of drug therapy. "How often have you done the procedure?" I asked.

"I do about five ablation procedures a week," he said.

Upon leaving his office, I realized the decision for opting in favor of the catheter ablation procedure would require *considerable* thought, as more questions cropped up in my mind while driving home. Is the procedure done in the hospital or outpatient clinic? How long is the stay? How long is the recovery period? What are the risks? Are there any side effects?

In order to learn more about the procedure, I did some research. I learned that the first catheter ablation on humans was performed in 1981 by Dr. Melvin Scheinman using high-energy direct current (DC) shocks. His work in this area, fortunately, led to the development of radiofrequency energy catheters, which, as described above, heat the catheter tip and perform much more precisely than the DC ablation. By the 1990s, radiofrequency energy catheters had replaced DC shocks. Dr. Melvin Mayer Scheinman was born on October 1, 1935, in New York City and grew up in Brooklyn. His father was born in Austria and moved to Germany, where the family was engaged in the shoe business. In the early 1930s, Melvin's grandfather realized what was happening in Germany and made plans for the family to leave for Israel, then Palestine. Melvin's mother was born in Poland. His parents met in the United States, where they married and had five children; Melvin was the fourth.

Dr. Scheinman earned his undergraduate degree at Johns Hopkins University and graduated first in his class. He continued his studies at Albert Einstein College of Medicine and graduated in the class of 1960. In 1965, he completed his residency at the University of North Carolina, Chapel Hill. In 1967, he was awarded a fellowship at University of California San Francisco Medical Center, where he continued his training in cardiology.

Travel, Family, Holidays and More Episodes

Thanksgiving Day arrived on November 23. We were spending the weekend at the Woodcliff Hotel, situated at the highest point in Monroe County in the Village of Fairport, New York. Joining us were a few out-of-town relatives from Syracuse, Buffalo, and Harrisburg, Pennsylvania. The hotel was close to the home of our son Kevin and daughter-in-law Tracy in Fairport.

Tom and I stopped over early that morning to help prepare the bird. After rinsing the twenty-pound Butterball turkey, I rubbed it with salt, pepper, sage, and butter. Then I lifted it into a roasting pan lined with sliced onions and chopped celery, covered it, and placed it in the oven at ten o'clock.

Afterward, Tom and I returned to the hotel with Kevin and our two granddaughters, where we all enjoyed the heated indoor swimming pool. Julia and Katie enjoyed tossing a huge beach ball to one another. We tried somersaulting underwater and standing on our hands, too, then we relaxed in the whirlpool hot tub for a few minutes before showering and getting dressed for dinner.

By 1:30 p.m., we all had arrived at Kevin and Tracy's for Thanksgiving dinner. Everyone pitched in, making it an easy day for all. My responsibility rested in bringing a five-pound bag of potatoes, boiling and mashing them to a perfectly smooth, light, airy consistency. I also made the gravy. Our nephew, Gary Haber, and his wife, Marcie, brought a homemade blueberry-raspberry pie and a pumpkin pie. Our son's in-laws, Diane and Gary S., brought homemade pecan pie and a bottle of Chardonnay. Tracy's Grandma Vicki, eighty-four years old, made a banana cake and her special butternut apple squash! Oh, yes, and that extraordinary stuffing, too!

Before dinner, we snacked on shrimp cocktail, crackers, and clam dip that Tracy made. Our three-year-old granddaughter, Julia, seemed to appreciate the value of healthy snacks and munched on carrots and apples.

After we were all seated in the dining room, Gary began with a prayer. Marcie mentioned that her family in Colorado always passed a lighted candle around the table as everyone thanked God for something personal and special. I would have liked to ask Tracy's Grandma Vicki to tell us about the first Thanksgiving she experienced in Brooklyn, New York, many years ago. But too often in life, we don't take time to reflect. At this time, I offered a prayer in remembrance of my mother, who had passed away the year before (Figure 15).

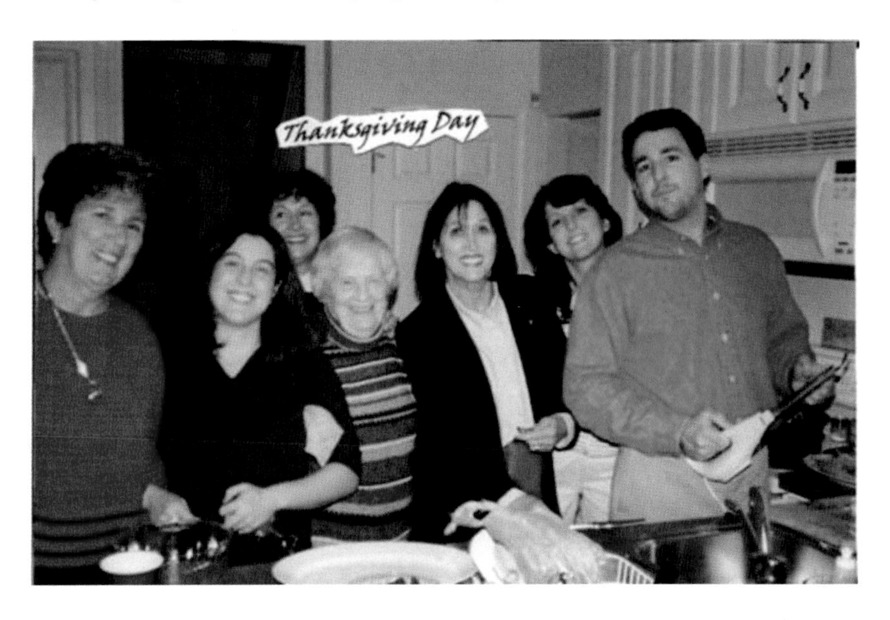

Figure 15. I celebrated Thanksgiving Day with my son's in-laws family in Fairport, New York. (l.to r.) Carol, Tracy, Diane, Grandma Vickie, Barbara (author), daughter Susan, and son Kevin.

Throughout dinner, we enjoyed delicious mashed potatoes, stuffing, cranberries, squash, sliced turkey, and lots of gravy. Topics of conversation included the undetermined results of the recent presidential election.

Gary managed to conclude that I voted for George W. Bush. Of course, he was shocked, especially when I elaborated that I was a long-standing registered Democrat who voted twice for Ronald Reagan and twice for George Bush, although the latter only won once. Like many, I was a Reagan Democrat.

We all laughed when Carol interrupted and reminded us of how Susan and her cousin Patrick as kids crawled under the dining room table and tape recorded our dinner conversation many Thanksgivings ago.

It was eight o'clock when Tom and I arrived back at the hotel, where we had a nightcap in the cocktail lounge before retiring to our room. Unfortunately, I experienced an all-night episode of PSVT, which kept me awake most of the night. Perhaps I had eaten too much turkey, or maybe it was the frenzy and excitement of the holiday! Thanksgiving, after all, had always been my favorite celebration of the year!

The next morning, the entire family gathered in the lobby to take advantage of the hotel amenities and admire the breathtaking beauty of the exquisitely decorated fifteen-foot Christmas tree. Most of us headed into Horizon's, the hotel dining room, with its fabulous panoramic view of the skyline to the west, and the Bristol Hills and the City of Rochester, New York. Everyone decided in favor of the breakfast buffet, which included a spectacular array of delectable pastries, French toast, sausage, bacon, hash browns, Irish oatmeal, omelets, and pancakes. Because of my all-night episode of tachycardia, however, which had not yet completely subsided, I settled for an English muffin and coffee.

Later, Gary, the doctor in the family, headed for a workout session in the exercise room. Kevin, and the two little girls, Julia and Katie, again enjoyed the swimming pool. Because I had the all-night episode of PSVT (rapid palpitations), Gary had advised me not to use the hot tub. When the episode finally subsided, however, I jumped into the swimming pool along with the others and managed to enjoy the benefits of the hot tub, as well. Julia put her feet in the hot tub and sat on the edge as I explained to her that one must be at least eight years old to get into the whirlpool hot tub, and she complied (Figures 16 and 17).

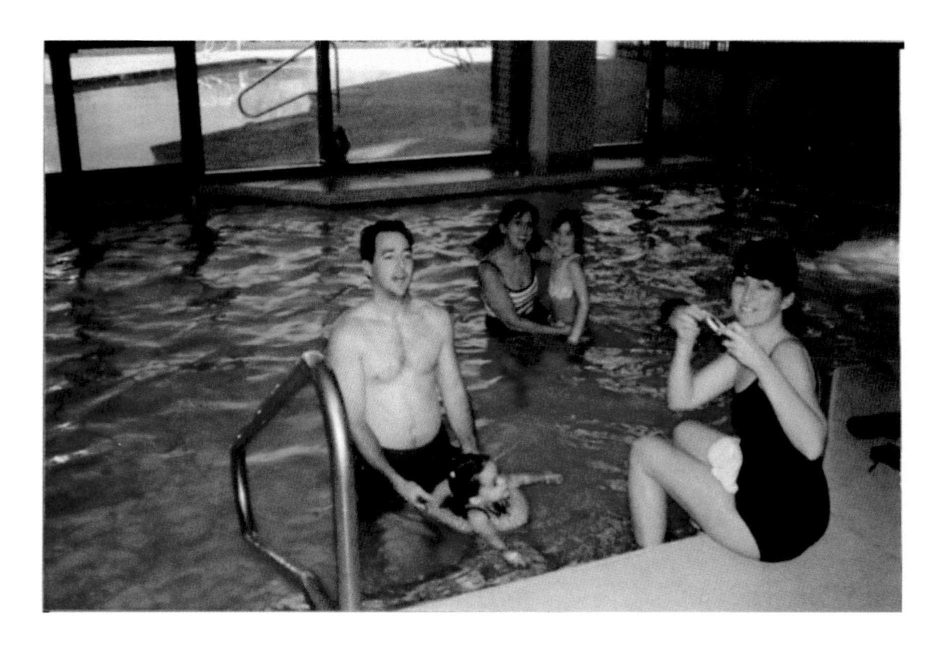

Figure 16. I enjoyed the indoor pool with my children and grandchildren.

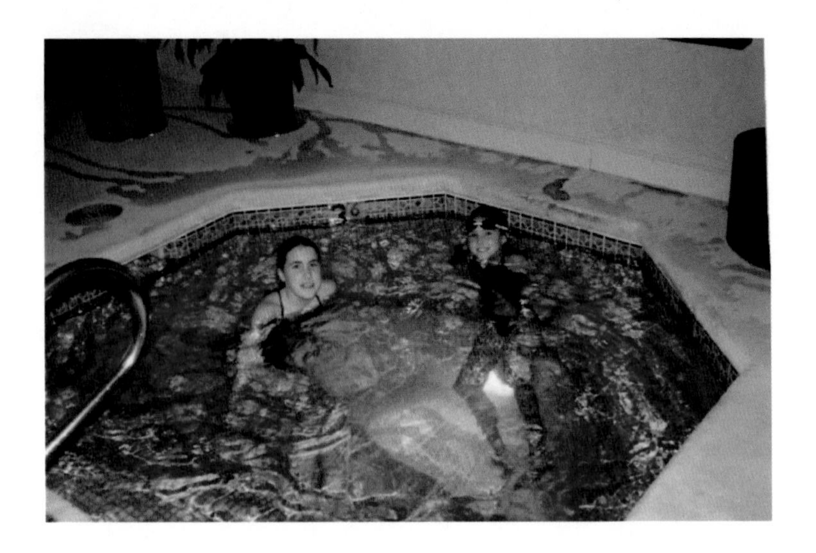

Figure 17. My granddaughters enjoyed the hot tub.

Upon checking out of the hotel, Tom and I stopped for an hour at Kevin and Tracy's, where they had prepared a care package of leftover turkey and trimmings for us to take home. Heading west on the New York State Thruway I-90 to exit 48A, we followed Route 77 through the back roads of Orleans and Niagara Counties to the City of Lockport, where we witnessed a beautiful sunset with alternating layers of pink and blue rising from the horizon toward the heavens.

Escalating Episodes and Rising Concerns

On Wednesday, February 7, I encountered my first episode of the New Year 2001. Crafts & Creations had an enormous collection of Valentine cards, door wreaths, fabrics, ribbon, wrapping paper, artificial flowers, and a variety of other items of interest on sale. The store was located only a few blocks from home, so I decided to drive over and see what they had. After selecting a few choice Valentine cards, I decided to buy a few scented candle tarts, as well. But which scents did I like best? Aha!

Frasier fir, oriental spice, apple crisp, freshly-cut roses, or kiwi berries. After enjoying a few quick, healthy sniffs of each, however—and at the same time inhaling more and more oxygen—I suddenly began feeling weak and faint. I felt my heart racing. I tried breathing in a normal fashion and in a few minutes, I began feeling better. I walked up to the counter, made a quick purchase, and headed out the door. Normal sinus rhythm did not occur immediately, but rather about an hour after I arrived home.

A week later, during my annual physical examination at the family doctor, I encountered a similar experience. I suddenly felt light-headed and faint after inhaling a few repeated deep breaths of oxygen at the doctor's request. Still seated on the examination table, I interrupted and cautioned him by explaining how I was feeling and added that I must have inhaled too much oxygen.

At that point, however, he corrected me and said, "No, you're getting too much carbon dioxide." He added that the normal breathing cycle rids the body of carbon dioxide and brings in fresh oxygen. Sniffing the scent of candles, however, is not normal breathing. When you take quick, shallow breaths, you risk hyperventilation. Light-headedness and dizziness are signs of hyperventilation and signal too much carbon dioxide in the body. Too much carbon dioxide can also bring on headaches and feeling tired. One needs to find fresh air to help rid the body of excess carbon dioxide.

Deep breathing had become part of a ritual I had developed for cleansing toxins from my bloodstream since 1995 when I read about it in a book titled *Unlimited Power* by Anthony Robbins. It wasn't uncommon for me to inhale while counting to three, holding my breath for a count of twelve, and then slowly exhaling while counting to six. I completed ten cycles of this breathing pattern, and later in the day, I repeated it. Unfortunately, it didn't occur to me at the time, but many years later, I began to wonder whether this breathing technique might have triggered some of my episodes.

In retrospect, I can only recall driving to work one morning while engaged in this deep breathing pattern. I suddenly began feeling faint, my heart palpitating rapidly, and I was forced to pull off the road and roll down the window. In a few minutes, I was able to continue driving to work. At this time, however, I did not relate deep breathing as possibly linked to tachycardia, as it had not triggered episodes in the past.

Since my cardiologist recommended and prescribed a beta-blocker in October, I had been taking it on a regular basis for four months. Many side effects can result from its use, but my main symptom had been feeling tired and less energetic, especially during the middle of the day.

It was around midnight on a cold February night in western New York when I decided to have a cup of hot chocolate before retiring, basically to warm up as the furnace thermostat was programmed to drop from seventy to sixty-seven degrees at eleven o'clock. I had been sitting at my computer practicing writing dialogue for an hour and a half, and not moving had left me chilled.

As usual, I was dressed in warm flannel pajamas. Nevertheless, as has occasionally happened in the past, my legs and feet remained cold throughout the night, and this sensation often interrupted my sleep. I remember awakening in the middle of the night feeling very chilly. My legs were shaking, not outwardly, but internally, as if the blood was attempting to chug along in quick short movements. The best way to describe it would be to say it felt like the insides of my legs were shivering. With electric heat thermostats upstairs, the bedroom, incidentally, was always well-heated overnight.

The condition described above is very reminiscent of the way I felt upon awakening from surgery after my hysterectomy four years earlier. To facilitate the circulation of blood at that time, my legs were wrapped in heated air cushions. Perhaps, I thought, I should consider acquiring this type of medical equipment for home use. At five o'clock in the morning, I decided to get up and use the lavatory. Then I pulled on a pair of wool socks. This physical activity increased my heart rate, and consequently the circulation of blood, for as soon as I got back in bed, my entire body started to warm up.

I thought about the beta-blocker I was taking and wondered whether it had anything to do with this. Although I was only taking the prescribed minimum dosage, my exercise-trained heart rate was typically low to begin with because I enjoyed walking and especially rollerblading on a regular basis. For this reason, I began thinking more seriously in favor of having the ablation procedure and eliminating the beta-blocker and its adverse effects altogether. When the beta-blocker was prescribed, I was told I would have no more episodes, but this had not been the case. It had failed to break the cycle of erratic electrical impulses.

Several weeks later, on March 11, our grandchildren Julia and Katie were visiting us one Sunday afternoon with their dad. They lived in Fairport, so it was just about an hour-and-twenty-minute drive west on I-90 to our house in Lockport. During their visit, I experienced an episode of tachycardia. Around four o'clock I suddenly began feeling very warm, tired, and weak. Beta-blockers help keep the heart rate lower than the usual 180 bpm during an otherwise typical episode. Consequently, I did not feel completely incapacitated as on other occasions before starting the beta-blocker Inderal.

Nevertheless, I debated going to a tennis league, scheduled Sunday nights at seven o'clock. It was my turn to drive, however, so I felt obligated and did not want to let my team down. They needed me as a player and a driver. Unfortunately, the episode persisted throughout the entire evening, and as a result, I didn't do very well on the tennis court. My performance was abysmal. Around 8:30 p.m. I began feeling slightly better, but not in the best condition to drive again, but I did. We left the tennis court at the same time. As I was driving home, I felt light-headed and nauseated.

Upon arriving home at about 9 o'clock, I took my beta-blocker and retired immediately. My blood pressure reading was 116/76, and my heart rate was now 82 bpm. Soon afterward, however, I developed chills and chest discomfort that interrupted my sleep until about 2:00 a.m.

In the morning after breakfast, I was feeling much better. My blood pressure was 99/64 and heart rate was 66 bpm. By eleven o'clock the readings were 142/87 and 57 bpm, respectively.

The biggest news in March was the stock market. It had been tanking. On the thirteenth, I moved the entire contents of my 403b retirement plan into a money market retirement fund within Fidelity. Incredible when you think the bears were predicting 6,000 for the NASDAQ a year and a half ago. Today, analysts are speculating that perhaps the bottom has been reached.

We were spending the last weekend in March with Susan and son-in-law Michael in Harrisburg. As usual, their girls were busy with school, swimming, and ballet. Colleen, who was nine years old, showed me a letter she received from Jan Brett, a well-known author of children's stories. The letter was written in response to one Colleen and her friend Laura had sent to Jan inquiring how to have their story, *The Case of the Golden Unicorn*, published.

Later that afternoon, I was sitting on their living room couch reading the book *I Spy* to my six-year-old granddaughter Caroline when I experienced a sudden feeling of irregularity in my heartbeat followed by rapid palpitations. As soon as I finished reading to her, I decided to lie down and rest. I talked myself into calming down and everything was fine. Amazingly, my brain heard this message, and it listened and obeyed, and my heart rate returned to normal sinus rhythm in a few minutes.

About a month *later* in early May, I was awakened from sleep at 12:30 a.m. I had been asleep for half an hour and was laying on my left side when I awoke, and rapid palpitations began immediately. In retrospect, I wondered whether the episode had occurred first and had awakened me. I managed to fall back asleep, despite the episode, while praying to St. Therese of Lisieux, "the Little

Flower," and repeating calming words to myself and asking for God's help. Scripture says *you have not because you ask not*. James 4:3 So, I asked. A few minutes later, I woke up again—this time with a normal heart rate.

There Goes My Heart

It was a dismal rainy morning in May. We decided to drive to Niagara Prime Outlets located on Military Road in Niagara Falls, New York, twenty miles west of Lockport. After shopping for almost two hours, I puddle-jumped across the wet parking lot through the pouring rain to meet Tom, as planned, for lunch at Red Lobster. It was one o'clock.

As soon as I sat down at the table, rapid palpitations commenced. Upon reviewing the lunch menu, and ignoring the onset of the episode, I ordered shrimp scampi, which included a Caesar salad and plenty of shrimp and rice. As usual, my husband ordered scallops. I didn't mention anything to him about the onset of tachycardia.

As planned beforehand, Tom had driven to the shopping mall, and I had agreed to drive home. While driving, however, I experienced some fatigue in my arms and pressure in my chest. Again, I didn't mention anything to Tom about this episode of PSVT until we arrived home, at which time I decided to lie down and rest from 2:30 to 4:30 p.m. Circumstances prevailed, however, and I noticed that my blood pressure had dropped to 99/55 with a pulse of 174. Without hesitation, I asked Tom to take me to the emergency department at our local hospital.

We arrived at the hospital shortly before five o'clock. I was taken immediately into a treatment room. After a nurse measured my blood pressure, she told me it was in the normal range. Blood work was done to check for hyperthyroidism, as it has been known to cause tachycardia. In addition, I had a chest x-ray to identify possible fluid, and an ECG was administered. Shortly afterward, I was hooked up to an IV saline solution, sometimes called a drip, whereby fluids in a clear plastic bag flow through a tube and into the body. Normal saline contains sodium and chlorine, which replaces lost fluids and prevents or corrects electrolyte imbalances. When the emergency department physician appeared on the scene, I saw the nurse draw his attention to the monitor screen, which I could not see because it was behind me. Then he said, "Yes, I saw that."

A few minutes later, the physician administered an injection of six milligrams adenosine, an anti-arrhythmic drug used to treat SVT. However, it failed to affect any response or positive reaction on my part. Consequently, at 5:45 p.m., about two minutes later, a second injection was administered, this time twelve milligrams, which prompted a good response, and my heart rate returned to normal. Sinus rhythm resumed. For some reason, I sensed that the wait time for my response was longer than expected (as I did not respond to the first injection), because shortly after all was said and done, I heard the doctor say to the two attending technicians or nurses, "Whew! I was ready to give up."

At seven o'clock, the physician returned to let me know that all test results were fine. "Your pulse and blood pressure are normal, and you are ready for discharge."

Before leaving, however, he looked at me and said, "You should never let an episode of SVT go beyond an hour, or you could go into heart failure." Then he added quickly. "You did the *right* thing coming here today!" He also mentioned the use of vagal techniques and gave me a few examples I might try at home to resolve the situation quickly. "Try dipping your face into ice cold water or coughing hard. You might try gagging yourself." I knew submerging your face in ice-cold water can tighten puffy, tired skin and certainly wake you up. But during an episode of SVT, any of the techniques he mentioned could, I imagine, jolt the central nervous system and cause the heart to return to sinus rhythm (Figures 18–25).

05/21/01 0041843 73110710 F
OSHEA BARBARA
62 LINDHURST DR 716-433-8609
LOCKPORT NY 805

PT NAME PT AGE MR#

GENERAL

TIME OF EXAM ____ : ____ [AM / PM] ROOM # Card. Wall

CONDITION ON ADMISSION ☐ GOOD ☒ FAIR ☐ POOR ☐ DOA

HX FROM ☒ PATIENT ☐ FAMILY ☐ CAREGIVER ☐ OTHER ____

ADDITIONAL HX : ☐ EMS ☐ POLICE ☐ OTHER ____

☒ NURSING ASSESSMENT REVIEWED ☐ OLD RECORDS ORDERED AND REVIEWED ☐ EMS / PRE-HOSPITAL RECORD REVIEWED

COMMENTS : ☐ NA ☐ OLD RECORDS ☐ ADD HX ____

CC : Light headed palpitations

HPI : 1] LOCATION OF PROBLEM : Chest

2] BEGAN WHEN ? 2° ____ 3] BEGAN WHILE : ____ 4] ONSET : ☐ GRADUAL ☐ SUDDEN

5] SX SEVERITY [1-10] : ONSET ____ MAX ____ NOW ____ 6] SX DURATION : ____ ☐ GONE ☐ STILL PRESENT ☐ OFF & ON

7] AGGRAVATED BY : ∅

8] RELIEVED BY : ∅

9] PRE-HOSPITAL TX : ☐ NONE ☐ OTC MEDICATION ☐ RX MEDICATION ☐ O2 ☐ IV ☐ CARDIAC MONITOR ____

10] ASSOCIATED SIGNS AND SYMPTOMS : ☐ NONE ☐ OTHER ____

11] OTHER HPI : ____

ROS : CHECK POSITIVE RESPONSES BACKSLASH NEGATIVE RESPONSES

CONSTIT ☐ FEVER ☐ CHILLS — CV ☐ CHEST PAIN ☐ IRREG HEARTBEAT — GU ☐ DYSURIA ☐ FREQUENCY — NEURO ☐ HEADACHE ☐ ALTERED LOC — HEM / LYMPH ☐ BLEEDING ☐ SWELLING

EYES ☐ BLUR VISION ☐ DRAINAGE — RESP ☐ SHORT OF BREATH ☐ COUGH — MS ☐ ↓↓ ROM ☐ MS PAIN — PSYCHE ☐ ANXIETY ☐ DEPRESSION — ALLER / IMM ☐ ITCHING ☐ HIVES

ENT ☐ COLD SX'S ☐ SORE THROAT — GI ☐ N / V / D ☐ ABD PAIN — SKIN ☐ RASH ☐ TRAUMA — ENDO ☐ WEAKNESS ☐ ↑↑ THIRST

OTHER : ____

COMMENTS : ____ ☐ ALL SYSTEMS REVIEWED AND NEGATIVE OR N/C

ALLERGIES : ☐ SEE NA ☒ NONE ____

MEDICATIONS : ☐ SEE NA ☐ NONE Inderal, Premarin

PAST MED HX : ☐ SEE NA ☐ W/O PREVIOUS HEALTH PROBLEMS

CV HX ☐ NO ☐ YES : ☐ ANGINA ☐ MI ☐ CAD ☐ ASCVD ☐ CHF ☐ HTN ☐ OTHER ____

PULMONARY HX ☐ NO ☐ YES : ☐ ASTHMA ☐ PNEUMONIA ☐ COPD ☐ OTHER ____

SURGICAL HX ☐ NO ☐ YES : ☐ APPEND ☐ CHOLE ☐ HYSTER ☐ CABG ☐ OTHER ____

NEURO HX ☐ NO ☐ YES : ☐ SEIZURE DISORDER ☐ CVA ☐ OTHER ____

ADD PMH ☐ NO ☐ YES : ☐ DM ☐ PSYCHE DISORDER ____

FAMILY HISTORY : ☐ SEE NA ☐ MI ☐ CAD ☐ ASCVD ☐ HTN ☐ DM ☐ OTHER ____

SOCIAL HISTORY : ☐ SEE NA ☐ SMOKER ____ PPD ☐ ETOH ____ / DAY ☐ OTHER ____

PHYSICAL EX : VS ☐ SEE NA ☐ WNL T 98 P 15 [☐ REG ☐ IRREG] R 16 BP 115 / 59 [SIT ____ / ____ STAND ____ / ____]

NL / ABN — CHECK AND DESCRIBE POSITIVE FINDINGS — BACKSLASH RELEVANT NEGATIVES

CONSTIT ☒ ☐ APPEARANCE ☐ ACUTE DISTRESS ☐ OBESE ☐ CACHECTIC ____

HEAD / FACE ☐ ☐ NC / AT ☐ TRAUMA ☐ SINUS TENDERNESS ____

EYES ☐ ☐ LIDS / CONJ ☐ LIDS / CONJ PALE ☐ ORBITAL EDEMA ____

☒ ☐ PERRLA ☐ UNEQUAL PUPILS ☐ UNREACTIVE PUPILS ____

ENT & MOUTH ☐ ☐ EAR / NOSE ☐ TM'S INJECTED ☐ NASAL DRAINAGE ____

☐ ☐ MOUTH / THROAT ☐ PARCHED ☐ LIPS / GUMS PALE ☐ TONSILS INJECTED ____

NECK ☒ ☐ INSPECT / PALP ☐ TENDER ☐ JVD ☐ TRACHEAL DEV ☐ SUBQ EMPHYSEMA ☐ ↓↓ ROM ____

☐ MENINGEAL SIGNS ☐ CERVICAL ADENOPATHY ____

☒ ☐ THYROID ☐ TENDER ☐ ENLARGED ____

RESP ☒ ☐ RESP EFFORT ☐ RESP DISTRESS ☐ ASSESS MUSCLE USE ☐ INTERCOSTAL RETRACTIONS ☐ SPLINTING

Figure 18. General admissions patient history

CV ☐ ☑ CARDIAC AUSC ☐ IRREG ☐ BRADY ☑ TACHY ☐ S3/S4 ☐ MURMUR ☐ RUB
160
☐ ☐ CARDIAC PALP ☐ CARDIOMEGALY ☐ DISPLACED PMI
☑ ☐ VASCULAR ☐ BRUIT ☐ ABSENT / DIM PULSE ☐ UNEQUAL PULSES ☐ PERIPHERAL EDEMA
☐ VARICOSITIES
GI ☑ ☐ ABDOMEN PALP ☐ TENDER ☐ GUARDING ☐ REBOUND ☐ RIGID ☐ MASS ☐ PULSATILE MASS
☑ ☐ LIVER / SPLEEN ☐ H/S-MEGALY ☐ RECTAL HEME +
☐ ☐ BOWEL SOUNDS ☐ HYPOACTIVE ☐ HYPERACTIVE ☐ ABSENT
MS ☐ ☐ DIGITS ☐ CYANOSIS ☐ CLUBBING
☐ ☐ JOINTS / MUSCLES ☐ JOINT PAIN / SWELLING / TENDERNESS ☐ ABN MUSCLE STRENGTH / TONE
☐ ABN GAIT
SKIN ☑ ☐ WARM / DRY ☐ HOT ☐ COLD ☐ DIAPHORETIC ☐ CLAMMY
☑ ☐ INSPECT / PALP ☐ ERYTHEMA ☐ PALLOR ☐ CYANOSIS ☐ RASH ☐ ↓↓ TURGOR
NEURO / PSYCHE ☑ ☐ CRANIAL N [2-12] ☐ ABN CRANIAL N EXAM
☑ ☐ SENSORY / MOTOR ☐ SENSORY DEFICIT ☐ MOTOR DEFICIT
☑ ☐ A / O TIMES 3 ☐ LETHARGIC ☐ CONFUSED ☐ DISORIENTED
☑ ☐ MOOD / AFFECT ☐ ANXIOUS ☐ AGITATED ☐ DEPRESSED ☐ FLAT AFFECT
ADDITIONAL FINDINGS / COMMENTS :

RE-EXAM / PROGRESS : TIME ___:___ VS ☐ SEE NA ☐ WNL T___ P___ [☐ REG ☐ IRREG] R___ BP___/___
PT CONDITION : ☐ UNCHANGED ☐ IMPROVED ☐ WORSENED ☐ OTHER

Adenocard 6 then 12 ē good response
Pt feels much better.

☐ CRITICAL CARE TIME : ___ MIN ☐ HX / PE LIMITED DUE TO :

ANCILLARY TESTS :

TESTS ORDERED — DOCUMENT ABNORMAL / PERTINENT RESULTS — * ☐ CHECK IF READ / INTERPRETED BY ER MD

☐ MONITOR ☐ NL ☐ ABN :
☑ EKG ☐ NL ☐ ABN : SVT 153, Axis 71, No ST-T ∆,
OLD EKG COMPARISON ? #2. NSR 74, PR 136, Axis 66 No Acute
☑ X - RAYS ☐ NL ☐ ABN : No Acute ∆
☐ PULSE OX ☐ NL ☐ ABN : O2 SAT___ [☐ RA ☐ ___ L/MIN] TIME ___:___
☑ CBC / DIFF ☐ NL ☐ ABN : WBC 8.3 HGB 13 HCT 40 SEGS___ BANDS___ LYMPHS___ MONOS___ EOS___
☑ BMP ☐ NL ☐ ABN : GLU 111 BUN 13 CR 0.9 NA 144 K 4.0 CL 108 CO2 23
☑ CMP ☐ NL ☐ ABN :
☐ U/A ☐ NL ☐ ABN : WBC___ RBC___ EPI___ BACTERIA___ DIP : CK 69 M.B / TnI 0.0.
ADD TESTS ☐ NL ☐ ABN :
COMMENTS :

ONSID DX: 1] SVT. 2] 3]
IAGNOSIS : 1] SVT Resolved 2] 3]
ID NOTIFICATION : ☑ PMD ☐ ON CALL PMD DR [illegible] @ ___:___ AM
DISCUSSION : ↑ inderal to 4x day.
☐ SPECIALIST DR @ ___:___ AM
DISCUSSION :

Figure 19. (continued).

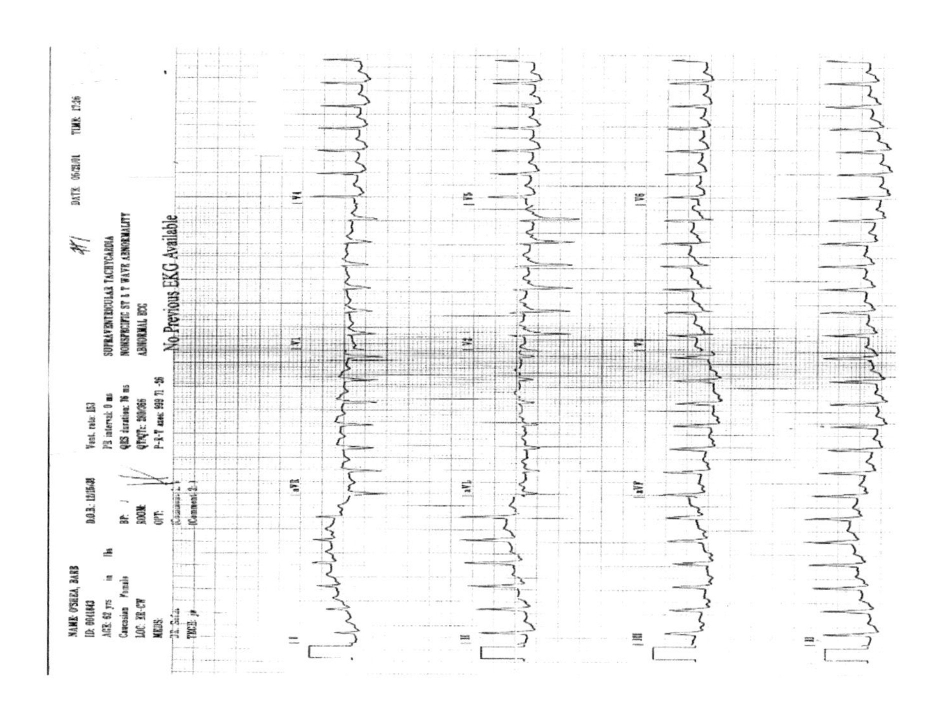

Figure 20. ECG testing report in the emergency department

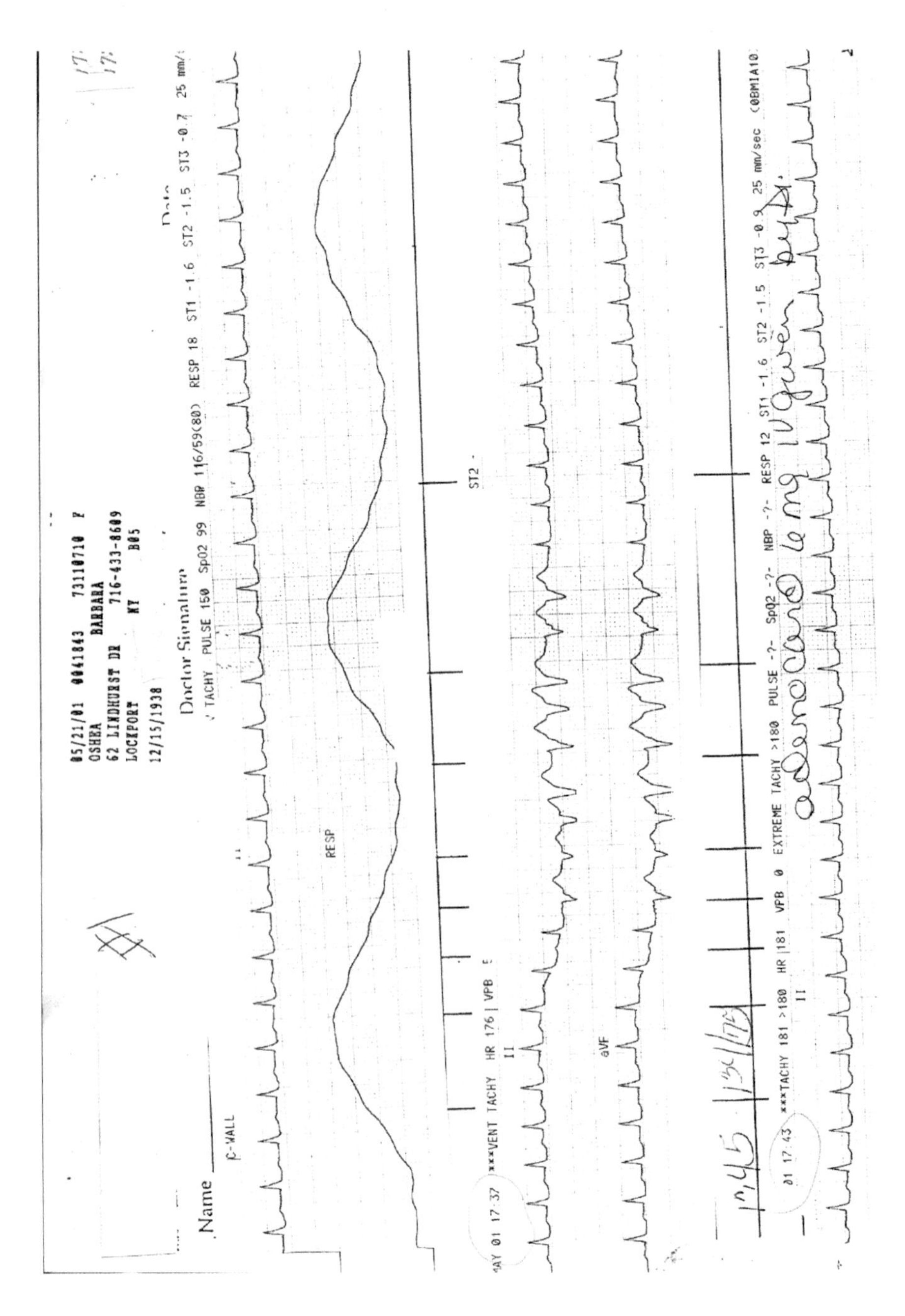

Figure 21. Further, ECG reports.

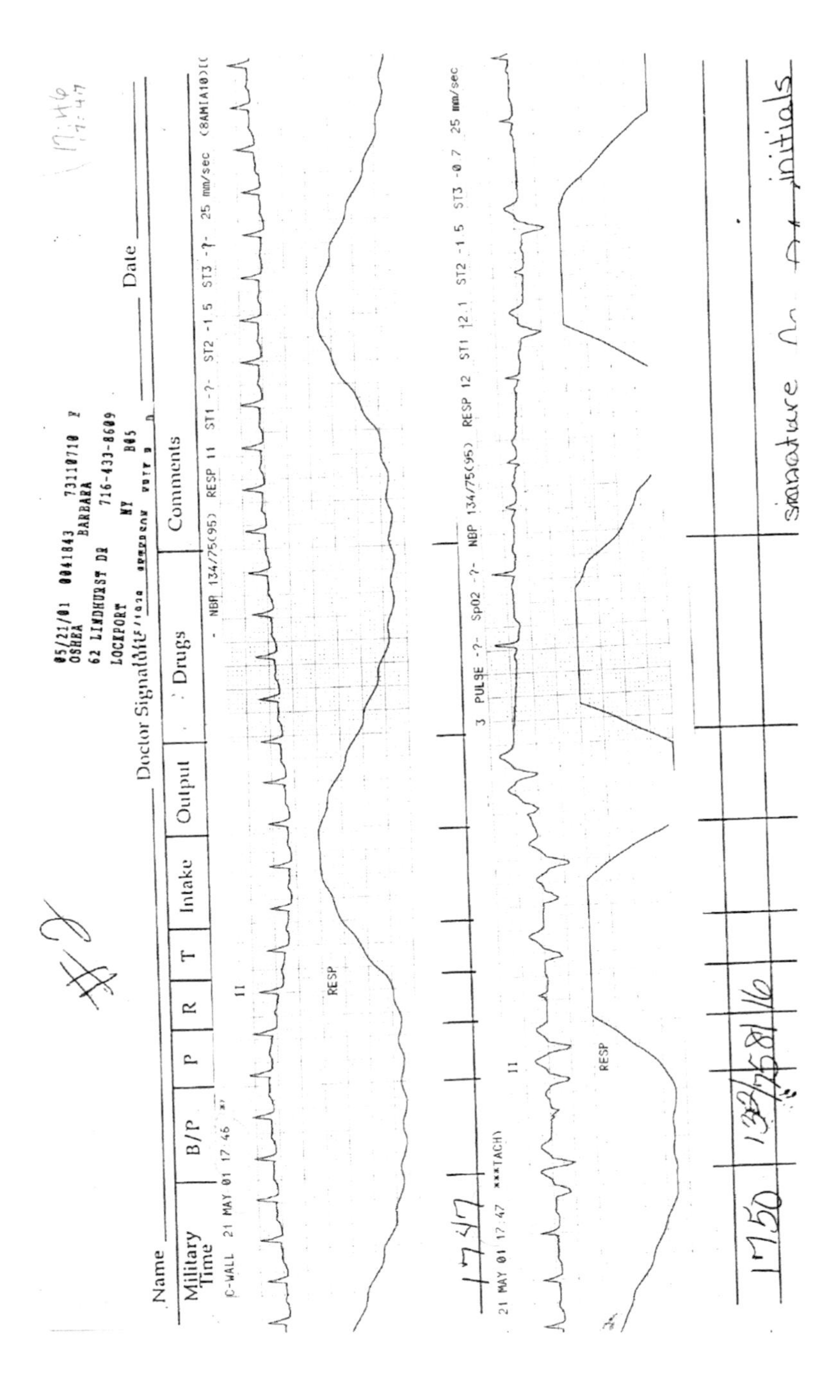

Figure 22. ECG testing continued throughout the emergency department visit.

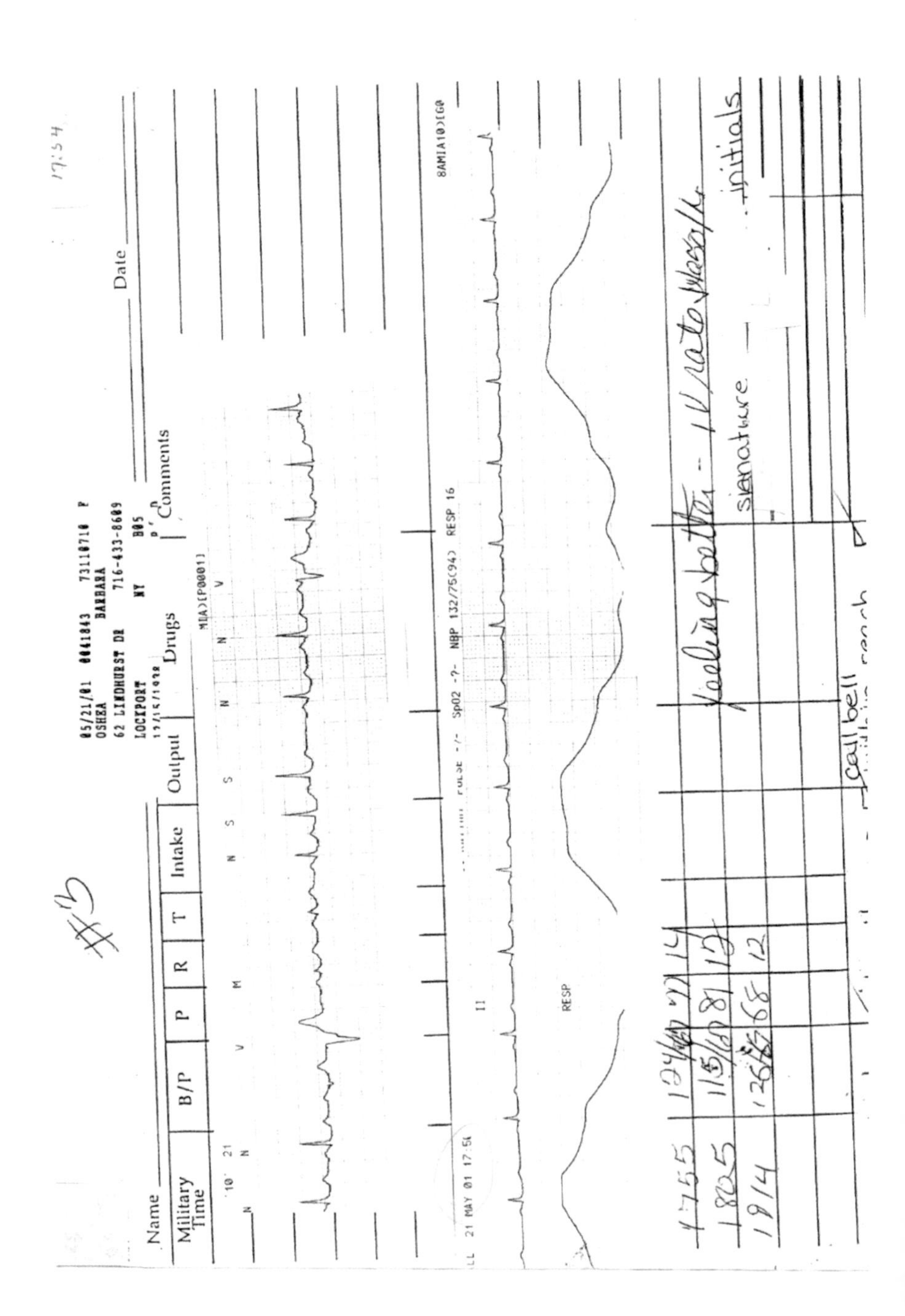

Figure 23. ECG monitoring continues.

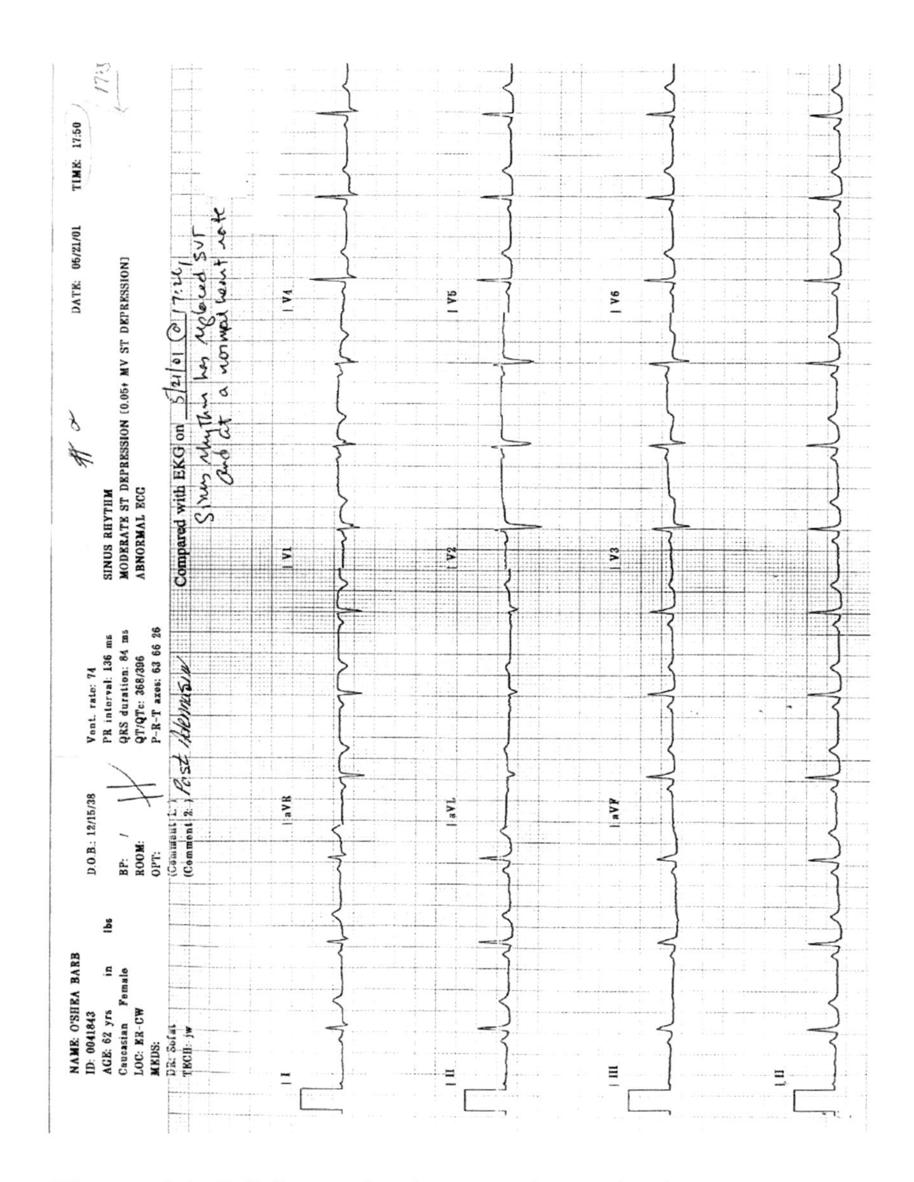

Figure 24. ECG monitoring continues in the emergency department.

NAME: OSHEA, BARBARA
AGE: 62 SEX: F DOB: 12/15/1938
COLLECTION DATE: 5/21/01 17:40 BY: DE

PATIENT ID: 73110710
ROOM: LMH ER

ACCESSION: 1141-LM0117 MR#:(

ACCESSION COMMENTS: # 1 CEP

TEST NAME	RESULT/FLAG	UNITS	REFERENCE
COMPREHENSIVE METABOLIC PANEL			
A/G RATIO	1.1		0.8-1.8
GLUCOSE	111 H	MG/DL	70-110
BUN	13	mg/DL	7-18
CREATININE	0.9	mg/DL	0.6-1.0
SODIUM	144	mmol/L	136-145
POTASSIUM	4.0	mmol/L	3.5-5.1
CHLORIDE	108 H	mmol/L	98-107
TCO2	25	mmol/L	21-32
CALCIUM	9.1	mg/DL	8.8-10.5
TOTAL PROTEIN	6.6 L	gm/DL	6.8-8.4
ALBUMIN	3.5	gm/DL	3.4-5.0
ALK PHOS	85	IU/L	50-136
AST (SGOT)	11 L	IU/L	15-37
ALT (SGPT)	30	IU/L	30-65
TOTAL BILIRUBIN	0.3	mg/DL	0.0-1.2
CARDIAC ENZYME PROFILE			
CPK	69	IU/L	21-232
CK-MB	1.2	U/L	0-6
RELATIVE INDEX - LMH	1.7		0.0 - 3.9
TROPONIN-I - LMH	0.00	NG/ML	0.00-0.60
CBC AUTOMATED W/5 PART DIFFERENTIAL			
WBC	8.3	10x^3/UL	4.8-11.0
RBC	4.25	10x^6/UL	4.20-5.40
HGB	13.0	GM/DL	12.0-16.0
HCT	40.2	%	37.0-47.0
MCV	94.5	fl	81.0-99.0
MCH	30.7	pg	27.0-31.0
MCHC	32.5	g/DL	32.0-36.0
RDW	13.3	%	11.5-14.5
PLT	232	10x^3/UL	130-400
MPV	10.8 H	fl	7.4-10.4
LYMPH%	41.0	%	23.0-52.0
MONO%	7.8	%	0.0-9.0
NEUTROPHIL %	43.9	%	33.0-76.0
EOSINOPHIL %	6.2 H	%	0.0-6.0
BASOPHIL %	1.1	%	0.0-2.0

ACCESSION/PROCEDURE	COMMENTS
TROPONIN-I - LMH	NON-AMI: TROPONIN-I < 0.6 GRAY ZONE: TROPONIN-I 0.6-1.49 AMI: TROPONIN-I >1.5

Figure 25. Results of blood tests

About nine o'clock the following evening, May 22, I encountered a brief episode of SVT. I was sitting at the dining room table with my laptop writing an ending to *The Green Hornet* for my memoirs. It was a story about an old jalopy my dad owned and had finally traded in for $75 toward a new 1950 Ford, for which he paid $1,600 in cash. As usual, I tried ignoring the episode and continued writing what I recollected about the day my dad took us to the dealership in Fredonia and bought the new car. However, the tachycardia soon distracted me from my work. I walked into the family room and checked the Weather Channel. The movement did nothing to alleviate the episode. Within a few minutes, however, I decided to try my emergency department doctor's home remedy suggestion and dipped my face into a large bowl of ice water. Amazingly, it worked immediately! At 9:45, the episode was over.

Summer Visits with Grandchildren

Since Tom and I retired two years ago, we've been taking more trips to Harrisburg. On July 12, during our summer visit with our daughter and family, we decided to take our granddaughters Colleen and Kelley home with us for a few days. The rest of the family would arrive a couple of days later for the weekend.

Colleen had fallen asleep on our family room couch that first night, so we awakened her at midnight, and we all climbed upstairs to bed. I slept with Colleen and Kelley in the king-sized bed in their mom's childhood bedroom. Wide awake now, we decided to play one round of "Guess Initials," during which Colleen promptly fell asleep. The initials I gave were N.O. (This referred to Nellie Olsen, a familiar fictional character from *Little House on the Prairie*. We had role-played characters from the book on Wednesday at the Radisson Hotel pool.) During the initials game, however, I experienced a mild episode of PSVT. It lasted only a half hour, and after it I fell asleep with no problems.

I wasn't superstitious, at least not at the conscious level, so I didn't think much about the fact that it was Friday the 13th. Our grandchildren enjoyed all the books, stereo/record player, games, and toys in our lower-level family room and outdoor recreation in our back yard. Tom and I took them to the gym at his school where he was principal. We rollerbladed, played with the scooters and ropes, and practiced shooting baskets. Of course, the Fun Fort outdoor equipment on the school grounds was the main attraction, and the girls enjoyed climbing it.

At bedtime, after this day of fun, *another* episode of tachycardia began, just like the previous night. This time, however, it lasted all night! Even when I went down to breakfast, the episode hadn't resolved. I managed to get some sleep during the night, but each time I woke up, I experienced uneasiness with pressure on my chest and rapid palpitations. I considered going to the emergency department again, but I was reluctant to awaken my husband at three o'clock in the morning.

Unable to sleep, I slipped out of bed and crept downstairs to the kitchen, where I filled the sink with ice cubes and water, into which I plunged my entire face. It didn't help. Knowing I couldn't sleep, I decided to wash the kitchen floor, after which I climbed the stairs and crawled back into bed.

It was not until Saturday morning when I started making breakfast pancakes and coffee that I began feeling much better. Sinus rhythm had resumed, and I was able to enjoy breakfast with my husband and granddaughters.

Upon awakening each morning, before getting out of bed, I routinely inhaled deeply ten times while holding my breath to the count of ten and exhaling slowly. At the same time, I stretched each leg one at a time, bending it at the knee, and bringing it up across my chest. After performing this stretching exercise, I felt ready, willing, and able to start the day, much like I did at age nineteen. In retrospect, I did not keep track of episodes occurring during any deep breathing or connect them in any way.

It was September 11, 2001. Around nine o'clock, I was working at the dining room table adding entries to my journal on my laptop when I heard the incredible earth-shocking news that a jet airliner had just crashed directly into the 120-story north tower of the World Trade Center in New York City. Within a few minutes, a second jetliner flew directly into the south tower. This prompted the Federal Aviation Administration to shut down all airports nationwide—unprecedented in our country's aviation history. Flights in progress were diverted to Mexico or Canada for grounding. Within minutes, a third (hijacked) plane hit the Pentagon. President Bush addressed the nation from Sarasota, Florida, where he was speaking at an elementary school. Osama bin Laden, who had made threats against the United States, became a prime suspect and was believed to be hiding out in Afghanistan.

Soon, a United Airlines jet crashed in Somerset, Pennsylvania. It was believed to be headed for a collision with Air Force One with President Bush on board. I witnessed most of this live on television. The United Nations headquarters was evacuated, followed by all government buildings. Names of the hijackers would be found by the FBI from passenger manifests. This event, fortunately, did not trigger an episode of tachycardia for me.

It was Wednesday, November 7. Four months had passed since I had experienced an episode of SVT. Apart from the major historical events in September that still dominated the news, my life was stress-free. On this day in early November, however, I awakened during the night with a rapid heart rate and pressure in my chest. I thought about gagging myself or trying one of the other home-remedies the emergency department physician had suggested in May. Fortunately, though, this was unnecessary, as the episode resolved quickly with the help of God, who consumed me with peace, love, and strength! Believing in the power of prayer as I did, I prayed a lot.

Thanksgiving 2001 and Another Episode

Upon checking into the Woodcliff Hotel in Fairport, New York, on Thanksgiving Eve, we were greeted by the familiar staff, whom we all knew by name, and they knew us. In fact, they always hung the Irish flag on the front lawn for Tom during every visit. I slept well through the night. I hadn't had an episode in three weeks.

That streak ended as soon as I awakened Thanksgiving morning when an episode of tachycardia ensued. It slowed me down considerably, making it almost impossible to get ready for breakfast in the hotel restaurant. Within a half hour or so, I thought it had converted to sinus rhythm, as I had regained enough strength to prepare myself for breakfast. "I think I'm ready to go down to breakfast with you now," I told my husband.

As Tom and I were riding down in the elevator to the lobby, however, I suddenly felt very weak again. As soon as the elevator door opened, I stepped out and sat down on the bench on my right. "Wait!" I told him. "I feel very weak and faint. I better sit here a while."

Our nephew, Dr. Gary Haber, happened to be in the lobby at the time and walked over to us. After explaining how I felt, he immediately tried taking my pulse but was unable to find it in my wrists. He finally succeeded when he placed his fingers over the carotid artery in my neck. He looked at his watch and counted the number of beats in ten seconds and multiplied it by six. "Your pulse is 160," he told me. At this point, he went upstairs with Tom to get my beta-blocker Inderal.

After I took the medicine, we were seated in the hotel restaurant, Horizons, the highest point in Monroe County, New York, overlooking the beautiful hills and vales, with the City of Rochester in the distance. About fifteen minutes later, Gary checked my pulse again and reported it at 80 bpm. By now, I was feeling much better and was able to enjoy an English muffin and a cup of decaffeinated coffee. The episode had lasted about two hours.

Episodes of PSVT were occurring more and more frequently. Rapid palpitations and pressure in my chest had again awakened me from sleep in the middle of the night on December 8. By now, I had learned much more about the ablation procedure and felt comfortable with the idea. Most convincing was the impressive success rate: 95 percent! Fortunately, I was able to talk myself out of that day's episode, again with God's help. By three o'clock my heart rate returned to sinus rhythm. My beta-blocker was not working to my advantage. Having the radiofrequency ablation procedure had become my top priority.

Will 2002 Be a Happy New Year?

Happy New Year 2002! During the month of January, I experienced two very brief episodes of tachycardia. Interestingly, both occurred at bedtime, just after I lay down to sleep. Both lasted only about ten minutes.

Again, during February, I had two brief episodes, both occurring as I crawled into bed for the night. Both lasted only about ten to fifteen minutes.

Three months passed without an episode of rapid palpitations. It was already Memorial Day 2002! I awoke on that bright Monday morning at about eight o'clock. Our room overlooked beautiful Lake Chautauqua, where we were renting a condo at Chautauqua Lake Estates in Dewitt, New York. Our guests—Gary, Marcie, Anneka, Carol Haber, and Elizabeth Grace—departed on Sunday after church after visiting with us since Friday (Figures 26-28).

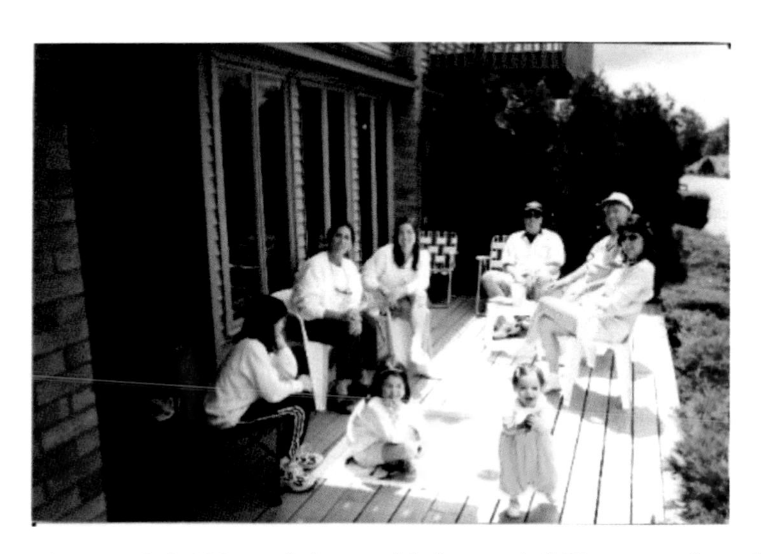

Figure 26. We celebrated Memorial Day weekend at Chautauqua Lake Estates in Dewitt, New York.

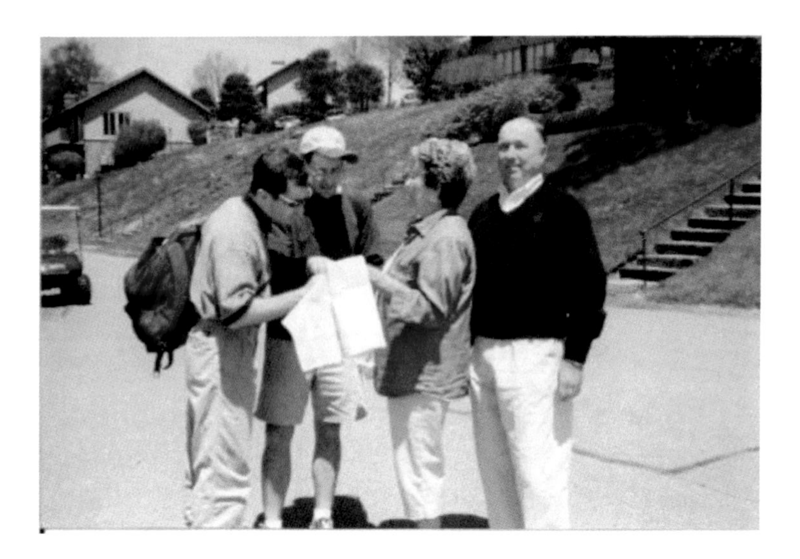

Figure 27. Weekend guests from Rochester and Syracuse, New York, study a map before departing.

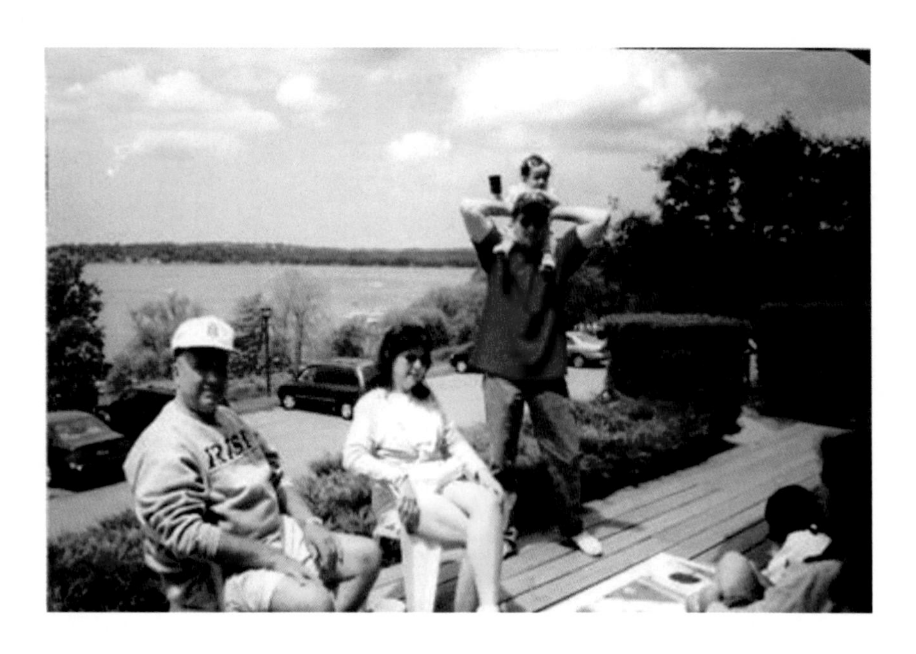

Figure 28. My husband, daughter, son, and granddaughter relax with family members on our deck overlooking Lake Chautauqua.

An episode of PSVT had awakened me earlier that morning. I tried to resolve the rapid palpitations and uneasiness with my usual calming thoughts, but that didn't work. I finally crawled out of bed and poured myself a cup of hot coffee and popped a piece of bread into the toaster. Eating breakfast didn't help much either. Tom had a golf date with Tom Harte, a friend from New York State Retired Teachers' Association who lived in nearby Lakewood. Before leaving, he turned on our cell phone and took it with him. I would call him if I needed help. The episode continued throughout most of the morning. I decided to lie down on the couch and watch a television program until eleven o'clock, which is about the time the episode terminated and Tom returned from the golf course.

Decision Regarding the Ablation Procedure

During a visit with my family doctor the following week, I expressed my view in favor of having the radiofrequency ablation procedure. However, I preferred having it done at the Cleveland Clinic and asked for a referral. He complied with my request and called the clinic to set up an appointment with an electrophysiologist.

US News & World Report had ranked the Cleveland Clinic as a top hospital for cardiology and heart surgery. Upon learning this, my decision regarding the ablation procedure was easy. At last, I felt comfortable and secure because of this unsolicited testimonial. In fact, I made a major life-changing decision that day!

It was late August. Driving west on I-90 at exit 177 near Cleveland, we took the Martin Luther King Parkway to Euclid Avenue, where we found the Cleveland Clinic Guest House just across the street from the clinic. After checking in, we walked across Euclid and down Clinic Drive, a divided block beautifully lined with grass, shrubs, and thousands of red, white, and pink flowers called impatiens (Figure 29). We entered the hospital lobby through a pair of automatic sliding glass doors. Once inside, we saw the gift shop on the left, and just beyond that, we were happy to find Registration Desk 15, where my journey would begin the next morning.

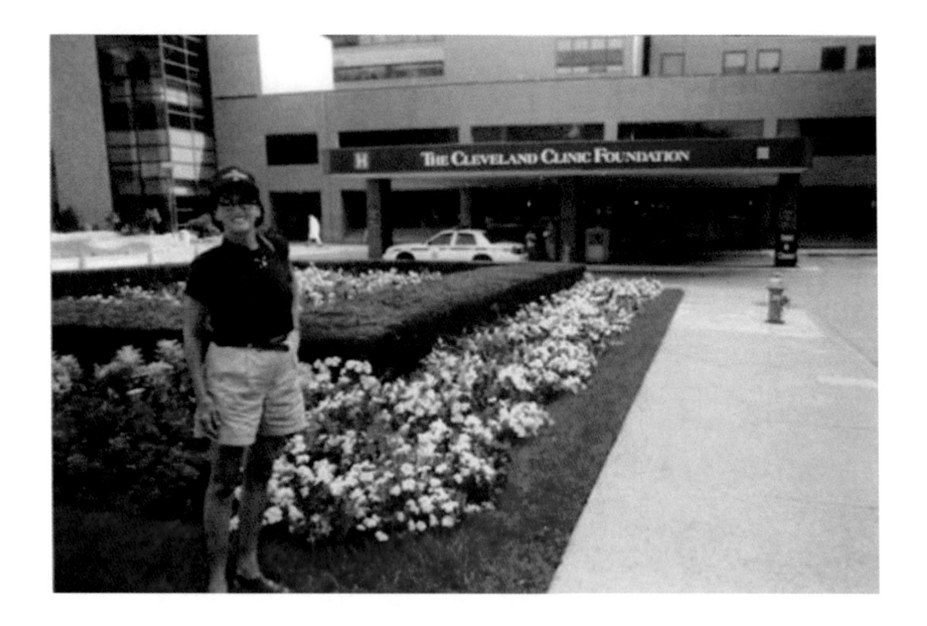

Figure 29. I arrive at the Cleveland Clinic.

While sitting outdoors on one of the wooden benches surrounding the fountain, we enjoyed breathing in the fresh air and marveled at the beautiful flower beds. We also enjoyed a fine meal in the hospital cafeteria. I was feeling comfortable about having the radiofrequency ablation procedure, which an electrophysiologist had explained to me.

"Although invasive, radiofrequency ablation is not a surgical procedure," my husband said, reminding me, "and you'll be in a sleeplike sedated state."

We didn't think or talk much about the electrode catheters, long, thin, flexible tubes placed into the veins in the groin. But I knew that radiofrequency energy heats the tip of the catheter, which is placed in the area of the heart causing the arrhythmia, and ablates, or destroys, the abnormal pathway. I was scheduled for the ablation procedure the next morning.

Having slept well through the entire night, I remained comfortable and relaxed when I arrived at the Registration Desk F-15 at seven o'clock the next morning. A physician assistant took my history, measured by weight, blood pressure, and pulse, and tested my reflexes—the works! Within a few minutes, the electrophysiologist stepped in to see me. He reviewed the details of the procedure related to various types of arrhythmia but particularly AV nodal re-entry PSVT with frequent non-sustained episodes with or without aberrance and subsequently sustained (as documented by my prior Holter monitor). He further explained that the rhythm then converts, in my case, from PSVT at a rate of about 190 bpm to atrial fibrillation with aberrant conduction and subsequent sinus rhythm resumed. He told us that the procedure would probably take place mid-afternoon.

We left the examination room and took the elevator to our next stop, where I had an ECG and four vials of blood drawn from the top of my thumb close to my wrist, the only visible vein. It was eleven o'clock when I began preparing for the ablation procedure. In a dressing room, I changed into a nightgown, pajama bottoms, and hospital slippers.

At this time, I was informed that two other patients were ahead of me. The lab technician drew another vial of blood and used a small amount to test for clotting ability. She told me that I scored very well: 1.0. My hand and arms were so cold that at first, she was unable to draw any blood at all, so she wrapped my arms in heated blankets. She inserted a twenty-gauge IV needle into each arm, one for sugar and water, which she started immediately, and the other to be ready when the sedative would be administered. Then I hopped into a wheelchair.

I wheeled myself to the waiting room as I pushed the IV cart along in front of me. Looking for Tom, I realized he had not yet returned from lunch. I seated myself next to an empty chair, where he joined me soon afterward. We kept busy reading *Newsweek*, *Irish America*, daily newspapers, and working on crossword puzzles throughout the afternoon. Headline stories centered on the West Nile mosquito virus, the sagging economy, deflation, and the question of whether our country would go to war in Iraq.

Around two o'clock my electrophysiologist spoke with us, explaining the delay. Others had moved ahead of me because I had been delayed by outpatient testing and evaluation all morning. I expressed concern about starting the procedure so late. He remarked that they took the older folks with more serious conditions first. When I asked whether it would be around three o'clock, he said, "No, it will be later."

An hour later, the doctor approached us again, but this time with the nurse-manager. They explained that the procedure most likely could begin at five o'clock at the earliest and that it would take three to four hours. They understood that I was uncomfortable with the timing and offered to reschedule the procedure for Monday, October 21. I would be first on the list, reporting at 6:30 a.m., and they assured me I wouldn't be bumped. They offered to buy us dinner in the hospital cafeteria and pay for our parking.

The nurse took me to the lab, where she removed the IV needles from my arm. She asked whether I had a headache from fasting since midnight; I told her I did, and she brought me an Advil and some orange juice. After changing into my street clothes, they gave me a voucher for $10. I was famished, so we had dinner in the hospital cafeteria. Many years ago, my psychology professor defined starvation as food deprivation for twenty-four hours. I could only agree wholeheartedly with that, for I was literally starving.

It was great being outdoors again near the circular fountain. We sat on a bench outside the main entrance, breathing in the fresh air, admiring the beautiful pink and white impatiens growing in thick massive clusters, and watching a flock of pigeons at our feet. A nine-year-old girl, enticing them with food, (which, of course, was probably not permitted), managed to capture three pigeons at one time and perched them on her shoulder, head, and arm. What a great picture that would have made. Visitors like us were enthralled by the sound of the splashing waterfall from the fountain, the chirping birds, and the smell of fresh flowers in full bloom. Some folks were reading, others meditating, and most were chatting on their cell phones. I kept busy updating my journal (Figures 30 and 31).

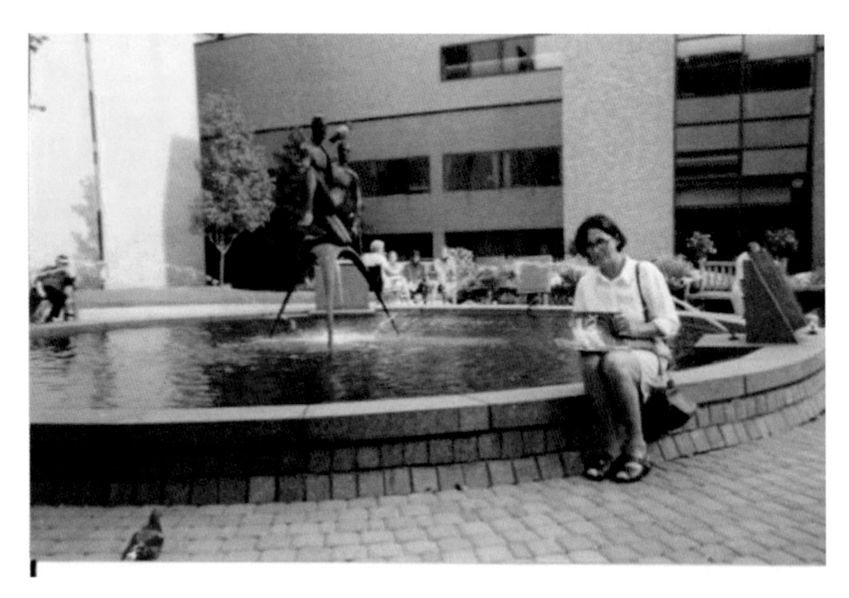

Figure 30. I enjoyed relaxing at the fountain on hospital grounds.

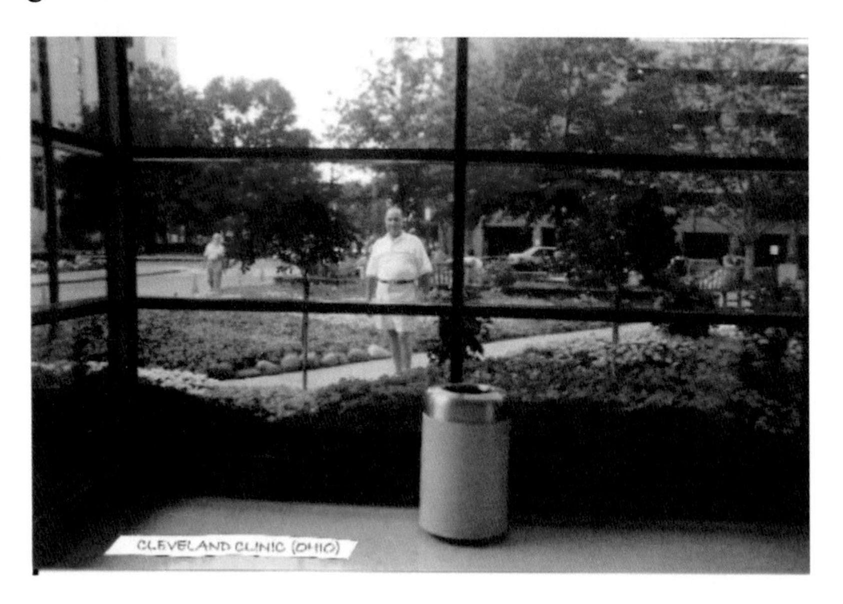

Figure 31. Tom is seen through the hospital lobby window while strolling the grounds.

As my husband and I attempted to cross Euclid Avenue, a lovely brilliant black woman in her mid-sixties speaking with scarcely any dialect difference exchanged a few words of caution about crossing this busy street safely. Our conversation continued as we crossed the street together asking her questions regarding directions. Following Euclid Avenue to the left, she told us, would lead downtown to Lake Erie and Jacobs Field, where a blimp was now hovering overhead.

When Tom asked her whether she had always lived in Cleveland, she began her story as we stood on the corner and chatted for ten or fifteen minutes more. She told us that her family left the cotton fields of Mississippi in 1953, where hard labor, poor working conditions, and minimum wages were rampant. Nevertheless, her dad had taught her that if you earned five pennies, *you keep two of them.* She recalled how, after working all week picking cotton, they spent Saturday night counting and sorting the pennies they stored in socks.

The family moved to Cleveland because it was perceived as a community of hard-working people, laborers, air-conditioned buildings, unions, and more importantly, non-segregated. The high school she attended in Mississippi was not equipped with typewriters, although the white schools were. Once in Cleveland, she enrolled in a typing class at a business school. Hired as a typist at General Electric, she continued to save a portion of every paycheck, as well as, take advantage of an employment opportunity investment program. The company matched this amount by 50 percent. She later bought five houses, became a landlord, then eventually sold them for profit. She gave us all the figures for each house, but only one stuck in my mind: a house she bought for $7,000 and sold for $80,000. She had recently bought a $300,000 home in Beechwood, a Jewish suburb of Cleveland. Before departing I said, "God bless you! Your story certainly represents a fine example of what the American dream is all about and how it really works!"

My Radiofrequency Ablation Procedure

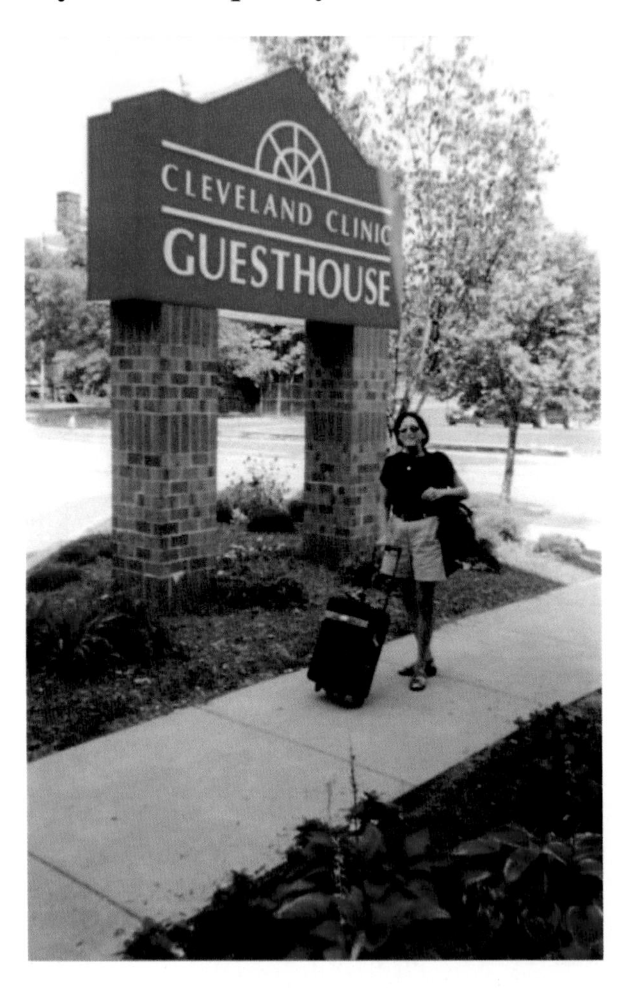

Figure 32. Checking into the Cleveland Clinic Guest House

Throughout the summer, I had managed to maintain normal sinus rhythm. Although some tachycardia might have occurred, it was nothing remarkable.

It was Sunday, October 21, when Tom and I returned to Cleveland, where we checked into the Cleveland Clinic Guest House, a hotel for patients and their families located across the street (Euclid Avenue) on the hospital grounds (Figure 32).

The morning of the procedure, I awoke at 3:30 a.m. with an exasperating episode of tachycardia. Of course, I could not get back to sleep. I wished that it was already 6:30, my scheduled arrival time at the Clinic. I was anxious to get it all behind me. I had done some deep-breathing exercises the previous evening to help me relax. The rapid palpitations continued until it was time for me to get up and shower at five o'clock. I felt weak as I stepped out of the shower and again as I took the elevator down to the lobby.

We took the shuttle to the Clinic, a five-minute, two-block ride. I held onto Tom's arm as we walked into the building and rode the elevator up to Desk F-26 in the main building. I was hoping this would be my final episode of PSVT for life. After registering, I sat in the waiting area with Tom for a few minutes.

Preparation for the procedure included changing into a gown and slippers and placing my belongings in an assigned locker. A nurse in the lab inserted an IV needle into the top of each hand where the only visible veins were located. Through these needles, she drew blood to check clotting ability, checked my vitals, and then attached the bag of sugar, water, and nutrients (electrolytes). She also measured my temperature, blood pressure, and weight, which was 132 pounds. After this, I wheeled the attached apparatus the short distance to the waiting room, where I sat with Tom until eight o'clock.

A nurse practitioner approached us and informed me that it was time to start the procedure. She reviewed the process briefly with my husband and me. Then she led me to a gurney, helped me onto it, and wheeled me into the electrophysiology lab, where television screens, heart monitors, blood pressure machines, and various other equipment lined the walls. I was introduced to one of the doctors, who asked me to sit on the x-ray table. Electric nodes were stuck onto my back and chest, and a camera was placed near me.

I said, "I experienced a lengthy episode of PSVT earlier this morning."

"Oh," replied the doctor, "that's a good thing! It will be easier to reactivate."

After asking me to lie down, the nurse began attaching the IV drug that would allow me to sleep during most of the procedure. The electrophysiologist must have entered the room sometime after I fell asleep because I did not see him until afterward. I remember waking up a couple of times during the procedure, but I was quickly put back to sleep. I recall waking up once to find a big transparent wrap – a type of airbag floating in space above my face. Someone (probably me) attempted to push it out of the way. Later, when I asked what it was, the doctor explained that it was part of the fluoroscope needed for taking pictures (Figure 33).

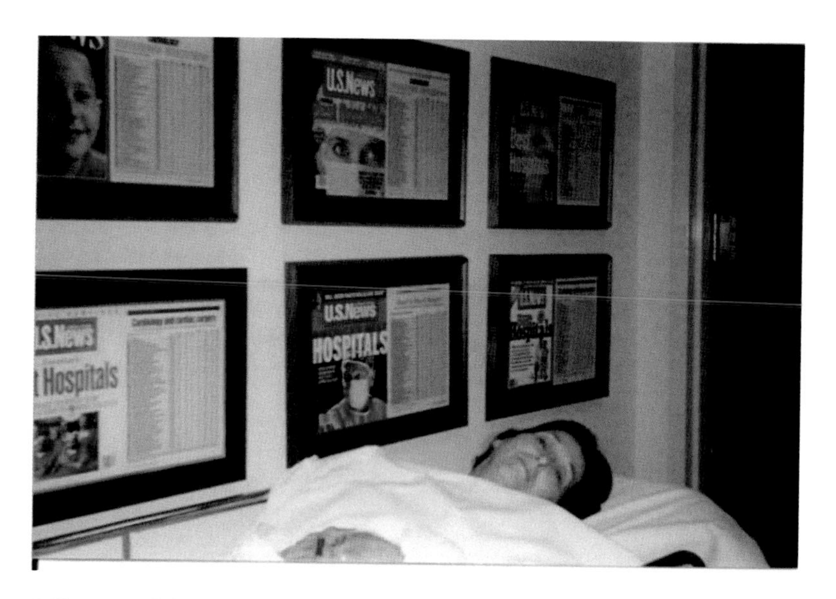

Figure 33. Recovering immediately after the procedure.

Soon afterward, I was surprised when I heard a voice say, "We're all done." I do not recall moving from the operating table (or x-ray table) to the gurney but was soon wheeled out of the electrophysiology lab into the hall. There I fully awakened and saw Tom and the doctor standing over me and talking. The doctor told us that they found only one area, ablated it, and found *no accessory pathways*.

Tom followed an aide who took me to private room M-10-53, where I was served a delicious lunch of mashed potatoes, roasted chicken breast, green beans, coffee, and a chocolate chip cookie, which I shared with Tom. By now he was hungry too, so he helped himself to some of my lunch. He stayed with me most of the time; the two times he left I fell into a deep sleep. My vitals were taken at 4:30 p.m.: blood pressure was 119/50 and pulse, 70. Tom walked with me up and down the corridor a few times for exercise. I carried a twenty-four-hour Holter monitor in my nightgown pocket.

I slept very well that night and woke early Tuesday morning with the six o'clock corridor noise but fell back into a sound sleep until 7:30. After breakfast, Tom arrived with the morning edition of the *Cleveland Plain Dealer*. After reading the paper, I showered and waited for the doctor to make his rounds and discharge me. "You could experience one more episode of SVT within a few weeks," he told me, "but no more after that." He smiled and added, "You can also discontinue the beta-blocker. In six weeks, you should have an ECG either at the Cleveland Clinic or with your family doctor." Before leaving he smiled assuredly and said, "You have a 95 percent success rate for a permanent cure."

A Change of Heart

At noon, Tom and I departed Cleveland and took the I-90 E home to Lockport, a 212-mile drive. It was warm, fifty-five degrees, partly cloudy with light winds, so we skipped visiting Presque Isle State Park in Erie, Pennsylvania.

"Instead," suggested my husband, "let's stop for lunch at the White Inn on Main Street in Fredonia."

"That's a good idea," I said. "We can eat outdoors on the front portico." It was a favorite spot of ours.

“How are you feeling?” he asked, during lunch.

“Really great! I know I’ll be fine now.”

While I was enduring the catheter ablation procedure on Monday, my identical twin sister, Liz, had traveled to Reading, Pennsylvania, from Shrewsbury with her daughter, Gretchen, and her eight-year-old granddaughter, Katie, where Katie had her first modeling job with the Boscov’s department store. Gretchen had called the offices a couple of months earlier asking where to send pictures and followed through with it. Although Liz had not experienced the same issues with SVT, she did have the radiofrequency ablation procedure in 2018 at a hospital in Baltimore to correct her episodes of A-Fib.

I later learned of two well-known persons who were also cured of tachycardia episodes after having the radiofrequency ablation procedure. Tony Blair, former prime minister of the United Kingdom, received in 2003 a diagnosis of SVT after fifteen years of intermittent episodes. In 2004, at age fifty-one, he underwent the procedure. Fay Weldon, novelist, and playwright, heard about him and followed by having the procedure the following year. She was seventy-four years old and had suffered frequent episodes of tachycardia throughout her life.

Knowing I would no longer experience another dreaded episode of PSVT, I could breathe more easily. Four days after the ablation procedure, Tom and I attended Grandparents’ Day at Brookside Elementary School in Fairport. Our granddaughter Julia had invited us to attend. We arrived at their house the evening before and stayed overnight. Julia's maternal grandparents joined us as we walked across the street and up the hill to the school. We met Julia's kindergarten teacher, Mrs. Fox. We enjoyed many activities, such as making handprints with blue paint, munching on snacks, and filling in worksheets listing our favorite color, sport, movie, food, and so on. Julia sat on my lap during the sing-along. What a delightful and relaxing day it was (Figures 34 and 35)!

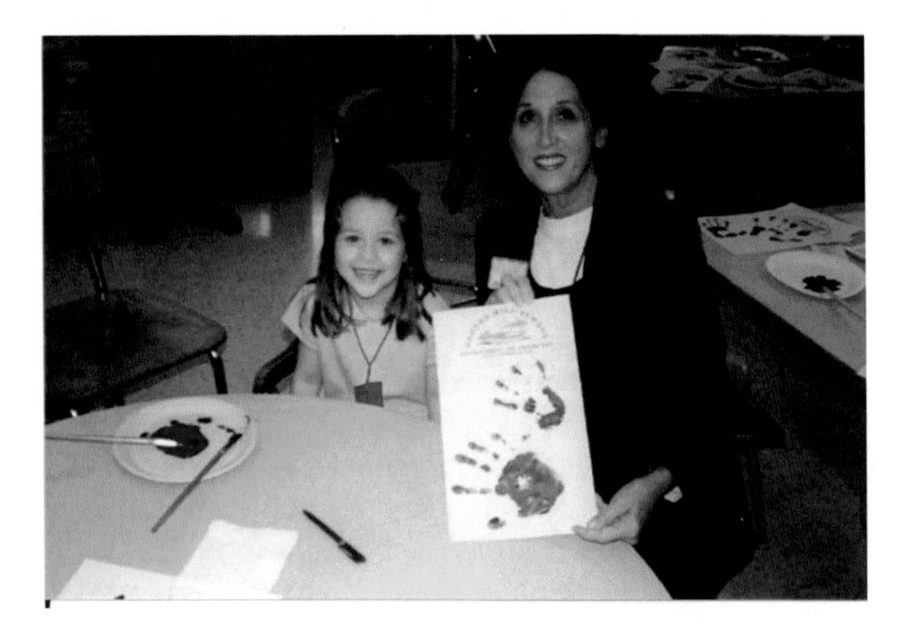

Figure 34. My granddaughter Julia O'Shea and I enjoyed making handprints with blue watercolor paint.

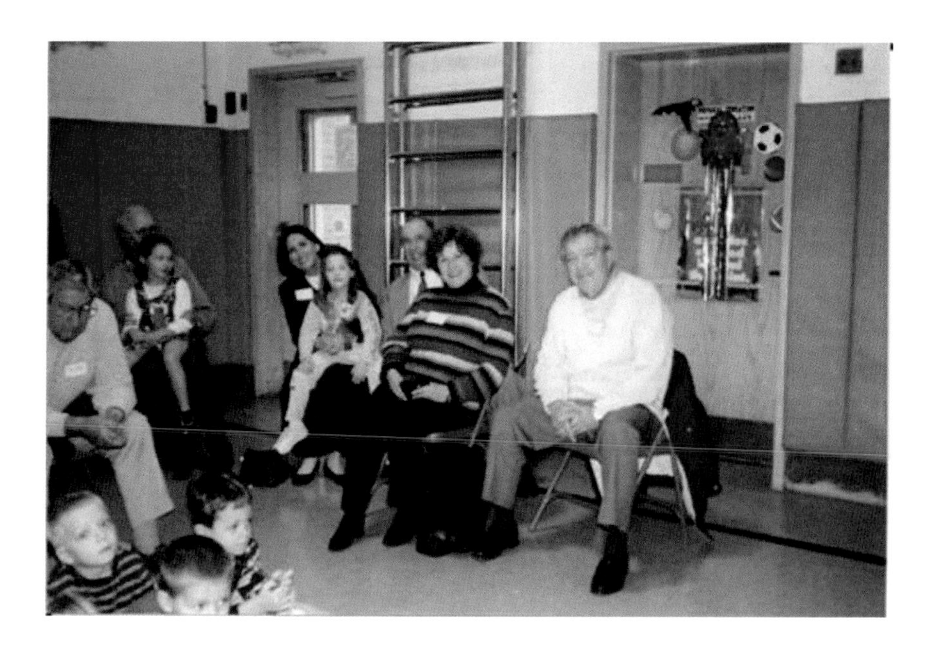

Figure 35. Tom and I attended Grandparents' Day at Brookside Elementary School in Fairport, New York.

Thanksgiving Day arrived again, but this year would be different. Having been cured of paroxysmal ventricular tachycardia episodes brought great relief to all of us! Upon greeting me at the door that day and knowing I recently had the ablation procedure, our nephew Gary (the doctor) asked, "How are you, Aunt Barbara?"

I grinned jokingly and replied, "I'm in *sinus rhythm*!" Amused and surprised by the unexpected use of specific medical terminology, he bent over with laughter.

As the family gathered in the kitchen just before dinner, we enjoyed munching on snacks and sharing our happiness with one another. We were prepared on this Thanksgiving Day to thank God for His many blessings!

Living with hundreds of episodes of paroxysmal SVT throughout the past fifty-five years of my life had not been easy. Episodes of PSVT were sporadic, unpredictable, and in my opinion, life-threatening. I had experienced fits of apprehension, uneasiness, fear, discomfort, anxiety, and distress, and I had been stricken with panic.

In contrast, life was easier now, more predictable and satisfying. I was delighted with the results of the radiofrequency ablation procedure and had discovered a new and wonderful feeling of *lightheartedness* in more than one way.

Now I was able to drive anywhere and enjoy life without interruptions—whether shopping, attending church services, driving, lying down to sleep at night, waking up in the morning or during the middle of the night, working at my computer, or standing in front of a class where, as a retired teacher, I was now substitute teaching in the Lockport School District. Because of the radiofrequency ablation procedure, I was finally *free* from this handicapping condition and able to function in the least restrictive manner—all thanks to Dr. Melvin Scheinman, whose work led to the first radiofrequency ablation procedure in the early 1990s.

Made in the USA
Coppell, TX
26 May 2024